FASHION
THAT CHANGED
THE WORLD

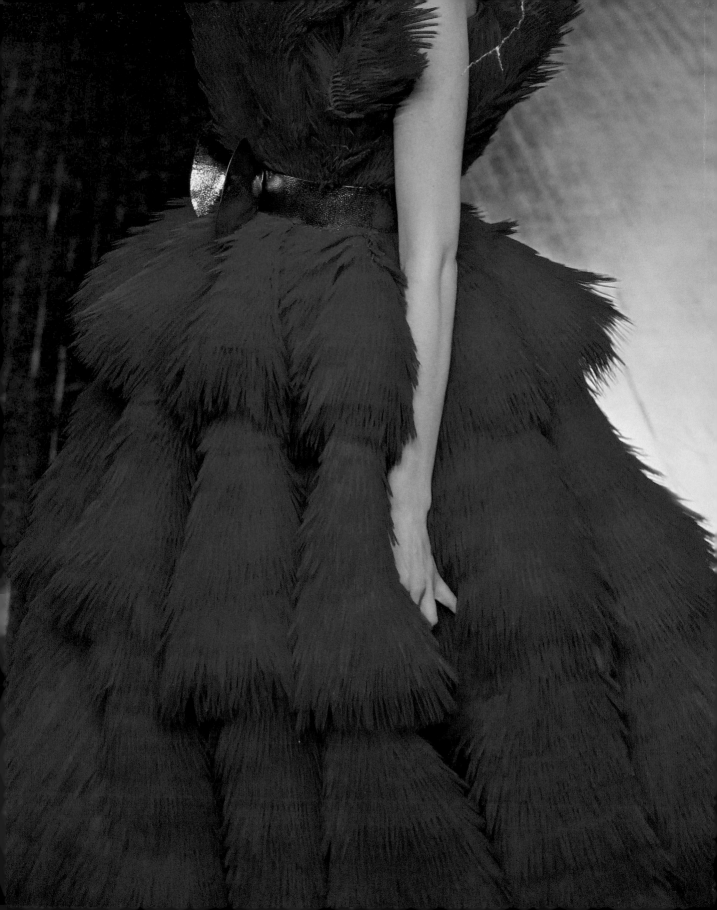

FASHION THAT CHANGED THE WORLD

Jennifer Croll

Prestel

Munich · London · New York

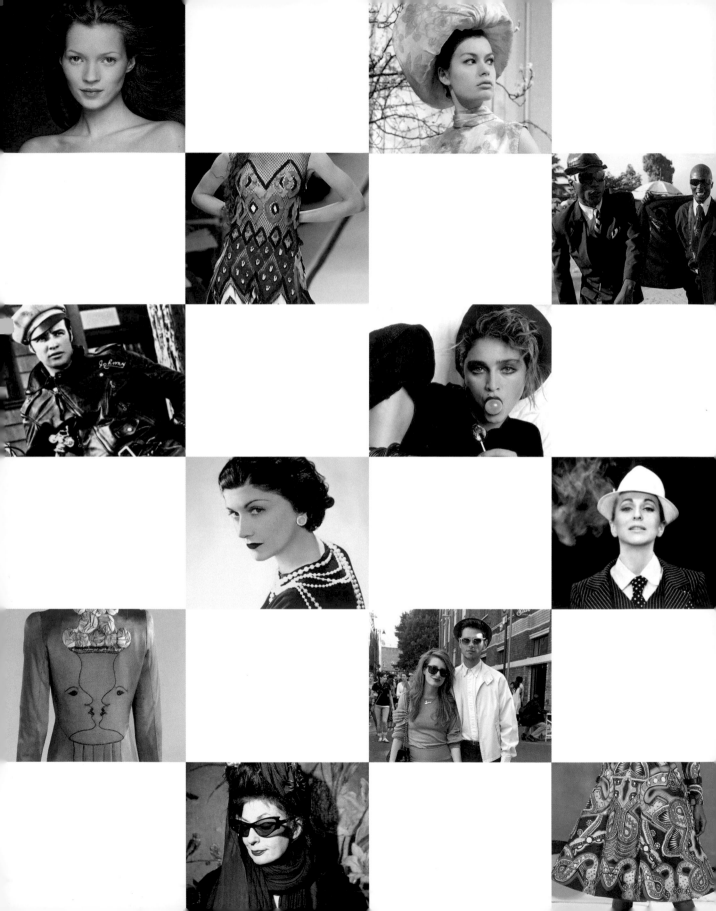

Contents

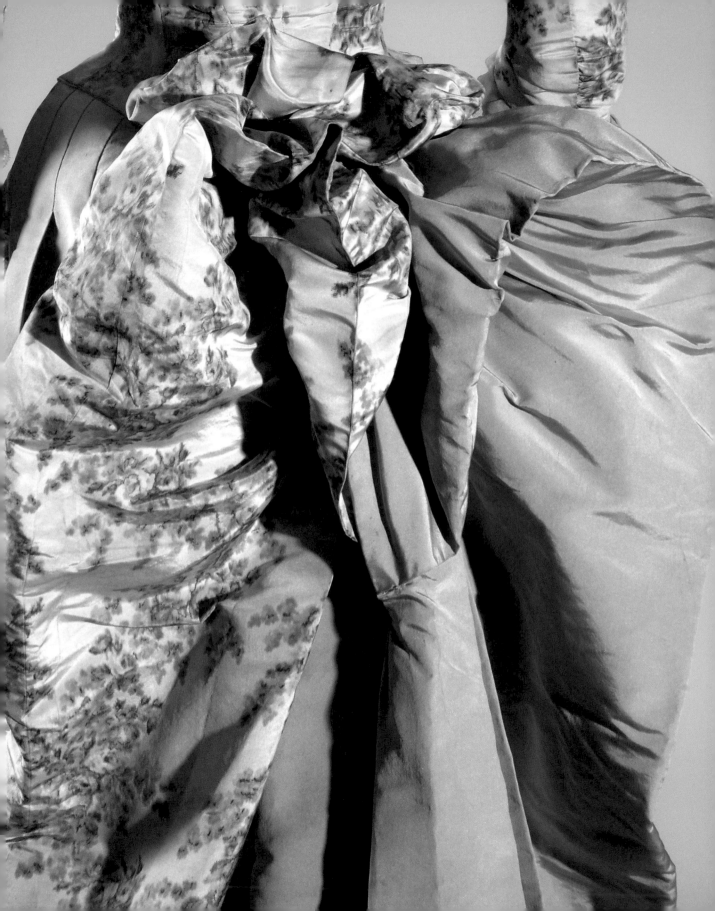

Introduction

Two people sitting in a café or restaurant, wittily speculating on the life stories of other patrons: it's a cinematic trope that may or may not be a real people-watching game. But it certainly has its basis in real life—we constantly make assumptions about who people are, what they do, and where they're from simply based on the way they dress. It's nothing new, either. Four hundred years ago, society's fashion biases prompted Shakespeare to include in *Hamlet* this piece of advice in Polonius's famous speech to his son Laertes: "Costly thy habit as thy purse can buy / But not expressed in fancy—rich, not gaudy / For the apparel oft proclaims the man." In other words: dress well, because people are going to judge you for it.

Of course, fashion choices are dictated by more than just the desire to look good. Our wardrobes reflect a lot about us: what country we live in, how much money we make, what society expects from us. In this way, it's easy to read history through fashion. As time passes, situations change: the world economy booms and busts, empires rise and fall, wars flare up, technology advances, culture becomes more or less conservative. All of these things affect the way people dress. Clothing becomes more or less ornate, uniforms turn into streetwear, trends spread at different speeds, hemlines rise and fall. Possibly more than any other cultural artifact, fashion is a sensitive measure of what's going on in society at the time, and a widely inclusive one, too—unlike art, which is only pursued by a few, or even democratic voting, which captures a disappointing percentage of public sentiment, fashion is a system that everybody takes part in. Everyone, after all, wears clothes.

But fashion isn't simply about blending in with the people around us; it's also about self-identity, and it's very much about choice. Beyond simply revealing who we are, fashion allows us to declare who we want to be. Through fashion, people rebel, challenge assumptions about their station in life, or traverse boundaries set by class, race, or gender, all by simply grabbing something different from the closet in the morning. Many fashion trends have sprung from individualistic or rebellious sartorial choices, and over time those trends have become the norm—giving future generations new ideals to either accept or reject.

Fashion That Changed the World digs into a multitude of social, economic, and cultural factors that have pushed fashion this way and that over the last few hundred years. Mostly covering the era from the Industrial Revolution onward, when the modern fashion industry took shape, this book considers a wide range of influences on fashion, including wars, sports, gender politics, media, culture, and entertainment. Over twenty concise chapters, it offers a historical snapshot of what we used to wear, and why we choose the clothes that we do today.

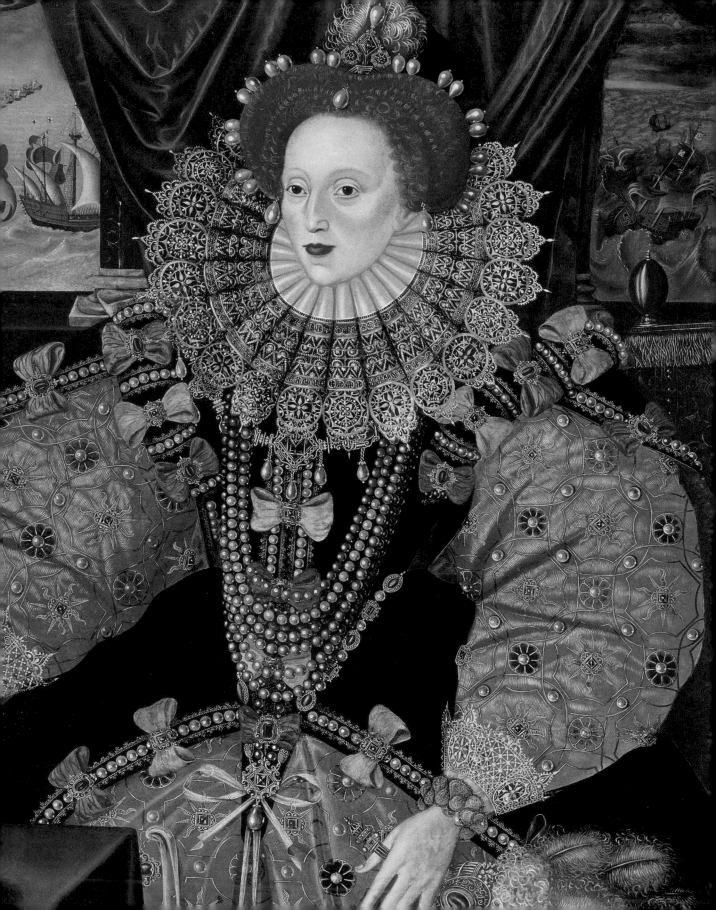

Royal Fashion

What Kate Wore is a popular blog dedicated to analyzing the fashion choices of Kate Middleton, the Duchess of Cambridge. Her stylish choices often mix high and low, equally representing couture and high-street fashion, a way of dressing that has won much public admiration. But Middleton is a departure from the past: these days, royals do their best to look like they're just one of us, but for most of history, royal fashion was beautiful, ostentatious, and the envy of common folk.

The first real queen of style was Elizabeth I. She crafted her look to cement her identity as the "Virgin Queen," with all its implications of youthful innocence. And, importantly, she didn't enforce the sumptuary laws barring her subjects from borrowing her style, meaning she spawned many imitators.

When she landed on the throne in 1558 at age twenty-five, during a period of political instability, Elizabeth was conservative in her dress, getting a feel for what would mollify the populace and what would enchant them. During her reign her style changed: she transitioned from simple cone-shaped skirts and embroidered sleeves to gowns with deep, revealing décolletage and farthingales (hoop skirts) accentuating her hips.

Elizabeth was, perhaps, the first fashionable redhead, and the ladies of England dyed their locks to match. She was also, by many accounts, extremely vain, and went to great lengths to avoid looking old. As she aged, she dyed her hair yellow or red to thicken and brighten it. Another of her tricks was a white makeup called "ceruse," which masked her wrinkles and made her appear delicately untouched by the sun. A mix of white lead and vinegar, ceruse certainly did give her face a fashionable pallor, but was also extremely toxic.

Her most significant fashion PR move was requiring all official portraits of her to be painted from a pre-established pattern—which became known as "The Mask of Youth." It served her purposes well: her image as a flame-haired, pale-faced young queen remains iconic today.

Half a century after Elizabeth's reign, Louis XIV ascended the throne in France. His seventy-two-year reign beginning in 1638 was known for many things: military conquest, the consolidation of power in the monarchy, and sheer longevity, but

left — Showcasing the queen's iconic red hair and flawless alabaster visage, George Gower's *The Armada Portrait* of circa 1588, when Elizabeth I was fifty-five years old, is a prime example of how the Mask of Youth kept her reputation young.

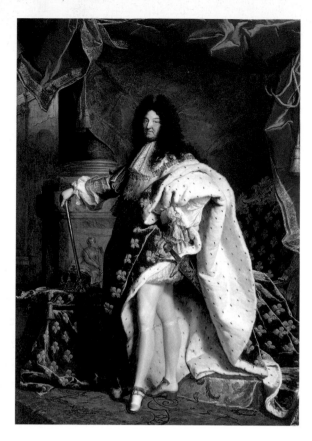

perhaps its longest-lasting legacies have been in fashion.

Louis XIV believed in the divine right of kings to power, and he dressed the part. He was a fan of large wigs and flashy jewelry, but his most notable achievements were in footwear. This may be partly because he liked to flaunt his legs, which he considered an asset. But there was also Louis's height; though there's no consensus, many historians suggest he was around five foot five, and high heels were an appealing choice for a diminutive monarch with a towering presence. During Louis's reign, he popularized everything from mules to stacked heels. Louis had an official shoemaker, Nicolas Lestage. Lestage charmed the king by designing for him a custom pair of golden silk pumps; the shoes fit, and so the relationship was born. At the time, there was a law requiring that shoemakers stamp their shoes with the mark of their shop—and so the brand name of Nicolas Lestage became incredibly well known, the forerunner to today's Jimmy Choos and Manolo Blahniks.

Another of Louis's influential decrees regarding footwear was that the heels of upper-class men's shoes had to be red. Of course we see contemporary echoes of that in Louboutins, a modern status marker. Louis's proclivity for dramatic and trend-setting fashions wasn't inherited by his immediate heir, but it was taken to a new level of provocation by his great-grandson Louis XVI's queen, Marie Antoinette. In 1770, at the age of fourteen, Marie Antoinette traveled to France from Austria to marry Louis XVI. She was taught how to style herself like a French queen, which appeared to be quite successful—until she found herself in a marriage with the curiously asexual Louis XVI.

above — The king of dressing for the part, Louis XIV points a toe and shows off his shapely gams in a pair of red-soled heels made to enhance his reputation, and his height, in Hyacinthe Rigaud's *Louis XIV of France* of 1701.

right — Louise Élisabeth Vigée Le Brun's Rococo portrait of 1778 shows the young Marie Antoinette in dramatic full panniers and a tall hairstyle, exemplary of the young queen's attention-grabbing style.

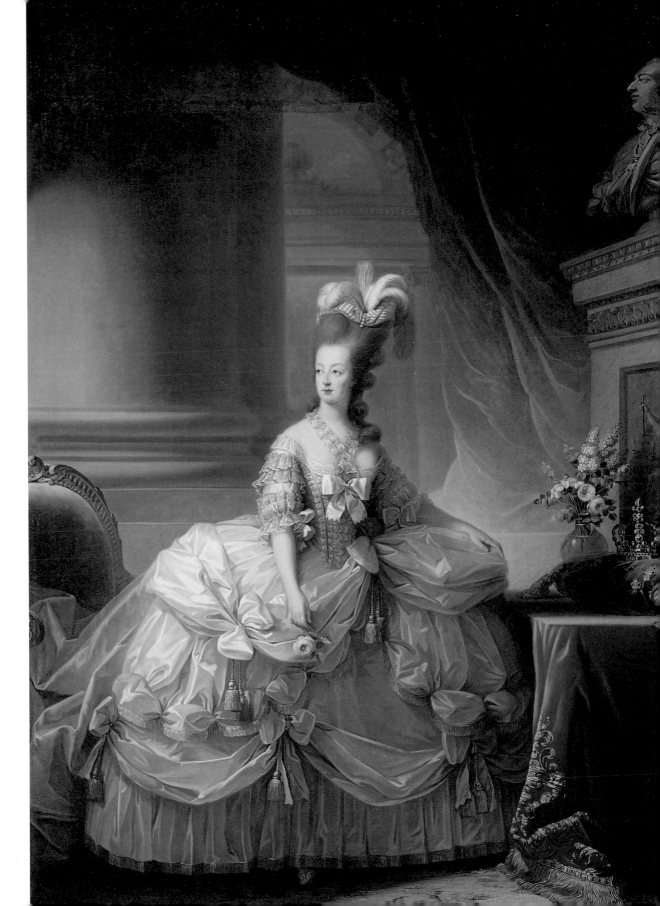

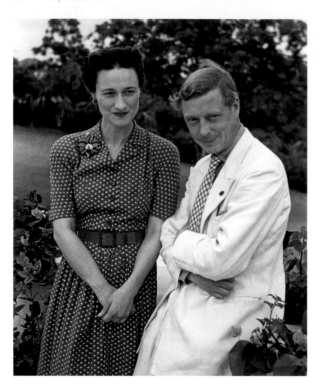

left — Controversy raged when Edward VIII abdicated the throne to marry twice-divorced Wallis Simpson; Simpson responded by dressing in a style that was beyond reproach.

At the time, the French queen's role was to bear an heir to the throne—little more. She usually wasn't a love match. Kings often kept mistresses who received generous allowances, dressed extravagantly, and in many ways outstripped the queen's power. But not Louis XVI. For the first seven years of his marriage to Marie Antoinette—four before they ascended the throne, and three after—their union remained unconsummated. Louis spent most of his time hunting and amusing himself, but never with women. Rumors about this unconventional marriage spread through France, and threatened to undermine Marie Antoinette's claim to the throne. And so she asserted her dominance in another way: namely, fashion.

One of her first acts of sartorial rebellion came on the back of a horse. In her copious free time, Marie Antoinette became an accomplished rider—and did away with the skirts typically worn by women on horseback, adopting men's slender breeches. And rather than riding sidesaddle, which was considered ladylike, she chose to straddle her horse.

But not all of Marie Antoinette's style decisions were quite so practical. Like the pouf, a towering construction made from wire and woven into the wearer's own hair with cloth, gauze, and horse hair, and then powdered white. This was then decorated with various symbolic items like small ships, animals, feathers, fruits, and flowers.

Marie Antoinette was responsible for popularizing the pouf with style-conscious Frenchwomen (much to the dismay of operagoers, who at one point petitioned to have the three-foot-tall headpieces banned from opera houses). Unlike her forebears, she didn't stay hidden away in Versailles; instead, she would make regular appearances in Paris to debut fashions, and in so doing introduced them to the public. Before long, the illustrations in French fashion plates and almanacs almost all resembled the queen. In another influential move, Marie Antoinette allowed her purveyors to keep their shops in Paris rather than just tending to her, as was the custom. This made it easy for them to keep tabs on trends as well as for Marie Antoinette to set them; she'd commission a dress or a hairstyle, and clients desperate to resemble the stylish queen would line up to buy it. Marie Antoinette explicitly okayed this, with a requisite two-week wait time before one of her

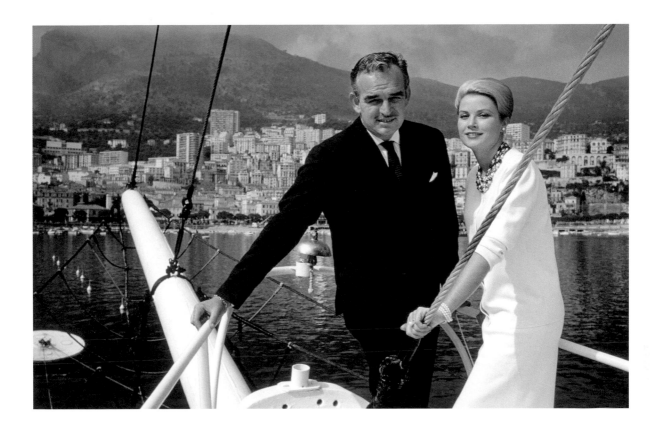

signature looks could be sold to the public at large. Exclusivity gone, regular people began to look much like the queen. But Marie Antoinette didn't just inspire the proletariat to dress like the bourgeoisie; controversially, she also inspired the nobility to dress like peasants. The country-girl attire that she wore at her palace annex, the Petit Trianon, triggered upper-class women to don the *gaulle*, a simple white dress made from muslin.

Marie Antoinette's capricious fashions were so inspirational and subversive that some credit them with provoking the French Revolution and guaranteeing the fall of the monarchy. What's undeniable is that she at once confirmed fashion's ability to assert and subvert power.

After the French Revolution, royal fashion was not what it once was: without ultimate power, royals had to adopt personas a little more in touch with their subjects. But that didn't mean they failed to inspire them. The nineteenth century saw a slew of fashionable royals, from Napoleon's wife, Eugénie de Montijo (see "Couture"), who revived the hoops skirts and corsets of the Rococo era; to Sisi, the sylphic Austrian queen with the punishing beauty regime; to Queen Victoria, who popularized the white wedding dress.

By the twentieth century, modern life brought some scandal into the lives of the British royal family. Wallis Simpson, a divorced American socialite, was the center of controversy when Edward VIII abdicated the throne to wed her in 1937; she reinforced her place by his side by dressing in impeccable style. More importantly, by the 1950s royals no longer sat solo on the pedestal of public admiration: they shared it with all of Hollywood. The picture truly blurred when Grace Kelly, a silver-screen icon, married Prince Rainier of Monaco in 1956. The new princess favored classic looks, such as tailored Chanel dresses. Hers was a reserved glamour. Her two trademarks were sunglasses and the Hermès bag that she used to hide her pregnancy; it was so

above — Hollywood actress Grace Kelly's marriage to Prince Rainier III of Monaco brought silver-screen glamour to the monarchy, at the same time lending the royals some pop culture relatability.

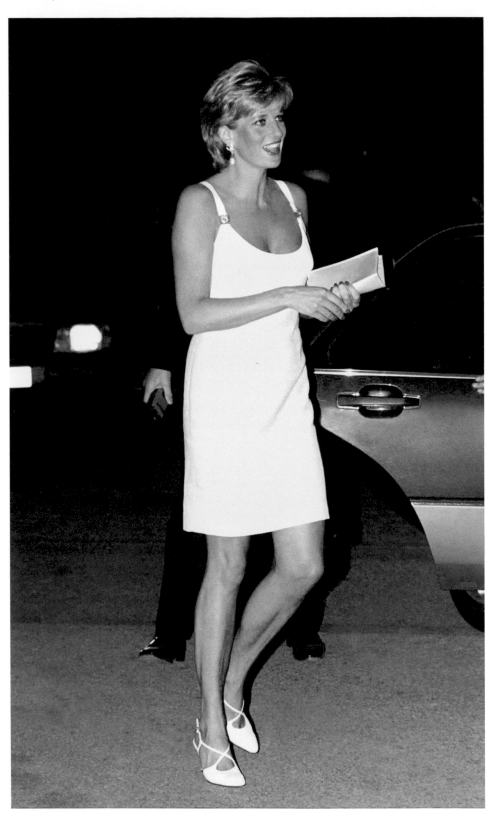

left — Figure-hugging Versace,
toned physique, and a defiant attitude: by 1995, at age thirty-four,
Princess Diana's style defined
self-reliant womanhood.

right — With an undeniable beauty grounded in middle-class values, Kate Middleton makes an off-the-rack Zara dress look like something fit for royalty (pictured here with her sister Pippa in 2011).

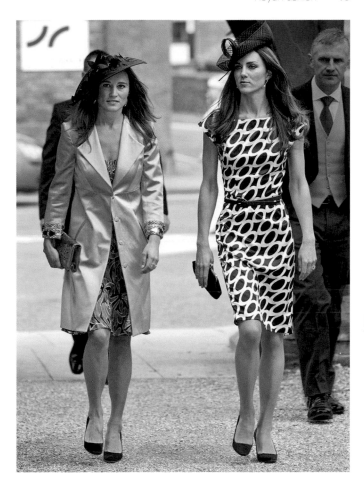

associated with her that it became known as the Kelly bag.

It was not until the 1980s that people truly related to a princess in Diana, Princess of Wales. After marrying Prince Charles in 1981, she stepped into a spotlight that was often harsh, but she was almost universally loved. Initially she wore a lot of gowns that were stereotypically "princessy," with full skirts and romantic styling, many made by Bellville Sassoon. But it wasn't until later, after her calamitous divorce from Charles, that she really defined her look: a short bob confidently swept out of her face (a style that caused hair gel sales to spike), simple lines, and clean tailoring—and a lot of sexy Versace numbers that showcased her athletic figure. Her look defined the aesthetic for a confident single woman, and she wore it until that fatal crash in the Parisian tunnel.

Now, in the middle of a financial downturn, when the institution of the monarchy is waning, it's perhaps unsurprising that we finally have a royal who embraces mass fashion and, by doing so, legitimizes it as glamorous. Before marrying Prince William in 2011, Kate Middleton lived a relatively middle-class life, and so was well acquainted with high-street shops. To the surprise of some, she continued to wear those affordable looks after entering public life. It was a wise move: it is easier for the monarchy to appear in touch with the people when it looks just like them. But Kate also inspires admiration for how she styles herself; on her, Top Shop comes off as elegant. Ever since women began to mimic Elizabeth I's red tresses, the sartorial line between royals and the rest has been blurring. Kate is the one to make it finally disappear.

Couture

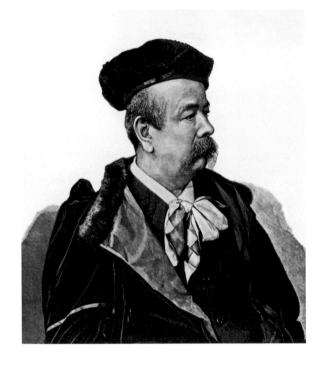

Rappers love couture, a fact that's well documented by songs like Kanye West's "Otis": "Couture level flow is never going on sale / Luxury rap, the Hermès of verses / Sophisticated ignorance, write my curses in cursive." Couture, of course, is the ultimate status marker: handmade, made-to-measure clothing that costs thousands of dollars isn't available to just anybody. But despite its hallowed reputation, couture's existence isn't a sure thing. In order to survive, couture depends on two things: a belief in the idea that clothes making is an art, and the presence of wealthy patrons, like Kanye, who can afford to buy it.

Couturiers may be celebrities today, but up until the late seventeenth century, designing clothes wasn't considered a particularly important profession, and was handled mostly by tailors. That changed during the reign of Marie Antoinette (see "Royal Fashion"), whose elaborate outfits made her *marchande de modes*, Rose Bertin, famous, though the designs themselves were a collaborative effort between Bertin, Marie Antoinette, and her court.

The first person to seize upon clothing as a means of individual creative expression was Charles Frederick Worth, who is consistently (and deservedly) referred to as the "father" of haute couture. His innovations paved the way for every couturier who came after him.

Born in 1825, Worth apprenticed for a draper and worked for a silk mercer before moving to Paris at age twenty, where he met his future wife, a shawl

above — Thanks, dad: pictured here in 1870, Charles Frederick Worth (known as the Father of Couture) introduced clothing design innovations that have shaped made-to-measure clothes to the present day.

right — New look, new everything: Christian Dior's hourglass silhouettes were the post-WWII era's fashion obsession. The designer is shown here, fitting a model in one of his creations.

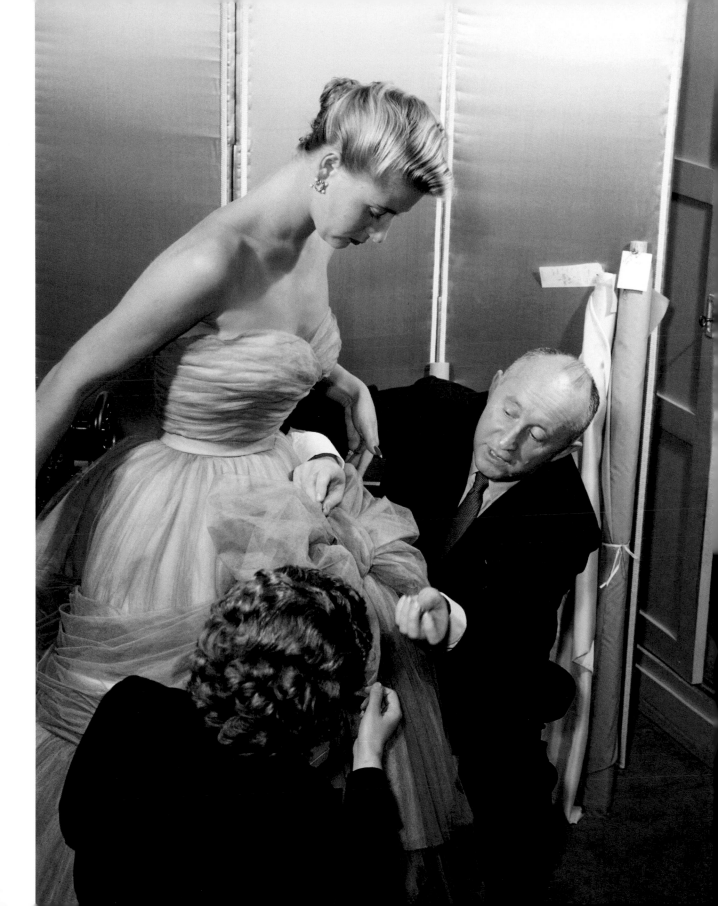

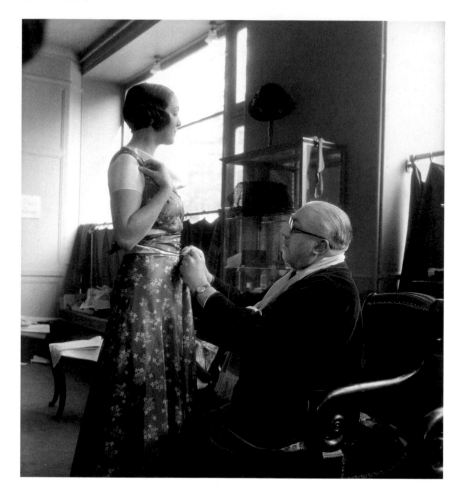

left — A rebel with a cause, Paul Poiret (shown here assisting a model with a fitting in the 1930s) aimed to revolutionize fashion with his antiestablishment ways.

model named Marie Vernet (see "Fashion Models"), when selling shawls for the upmarket silk mercer Gagelin. Worth began to design dresses to complement Marie's shawls, and it wasn't long before customers were ordering his dresses. The dresses Worth made at Gagelin earned medals, and by 1858 he branched off into his own business.

Unlike other dressmakers, Worth designed like an auteur: fashion was about what *he* wanted. Women came by appointment and trusted themselves to his taste, rather than commissioning theirs. Fortunately, Worth's taste was excellent, and the connections he had with the textile industry gave him access to the best and most interesting fabrics. Most of Worth's fashion innovations advocated simplicity and elegance; he got rid of the so-called cage crinoline, a massive metal lattice that supported a skirt, and made shapes sleeker and less fussy. His creations

were superbly tailored, flattering, and influential— so much so that in 1868 he founded the Chambre syndicale de la confection et de la couture pour dames et fillettes (later renamed the Chambre syndicale de la haute couture), an organization designed to handle labor issues and combat the copying of fashion designs.

Marie's modeling was instrumental to Worth's success: he designed for her and she marketed his creations by wearing them. Early in his career she snagged Empress Eugénie (Napoleon's wife) as a client, which was all Worth needed to cement himself as Paris's most important designer. Worth's team of seamstresses worked hard to keep up with the demand—only possible due to the innovations in sewing machines. By the early 1870s, he employed a staff of 1,200. He did, however, see some big competition, mostly from Madame Paquin, who also goes

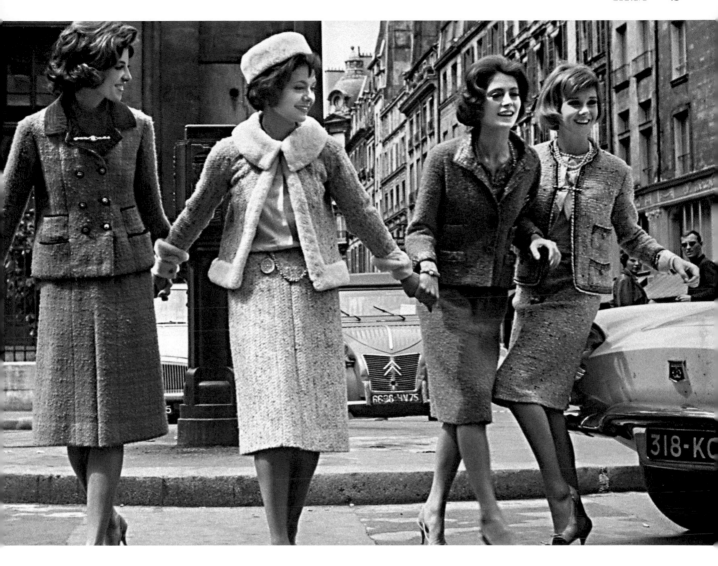

down in the records as the first female couturier. Her business was immensely profitable, and she went head-to-head with Worth in foreign sales. Worth may have founded couture, but it didn't really have any attitude until a young rebel by the name of Paul Poiret appeared. Poiret's designs flew in the face of convention. A true nonconformist, he wanted to turn everything upside down. Like Worth, his

above — Practical and elegant, Coco Chanel's designs—like these tailored suits shown in 1960 Paris—were meant for modern women on the move.

attitudes to fashion were shaped by his wife, a very slender woman whose lithe body was the antithesis of that era's voluptuous norm. The sleek outline he created using a corset that freed the waist but hugged the hips was nicknamed called "le vague" for its imprecise definition of the figure. By 1910 his bad reputation peaked when the pope condemned his "hobble skirt," which only allowed women to walk in extremely short steps. The controversy was excellent publicity for Poiret, who enjoyed the bump in sales.

Another invention of Poiret's was the traveling fashion show, which he took around Europe and to the United States. While in the US, he discovered that stores were selling copies of his work without his permission, which led to him create (with Philippe Ortiz of *Vogue*) an organization called Le syndicat de défense de la grande couture française, which pursued copyright violations.

Unfortunately, Poiret's over-the-top aesthetics didn't fly after World War I, and unable to adapt, he drifted into obscurity.

Interwar practicality nurtured the development of one of the century's most important fashion figures: Coco Chanel. A tomboy herself, Chanel's fashions were often inspired by menswear—revolutionary, at the time. She began designing hats, and from there moved into womenswear, opening her couture shop in 1919. Her clothes equipped women for lives on the move—appealing in the wake of WWI, when women found themselves doing what was traditionally thought of as men's work. She designed sweaters, jackets, and other mannish items with the essence of simplicity: no frills, no flourishes. Chanel's couture shop became extremely successful, peaking during the thirties and forties. Then she found a rival in Elsa Schiaparelli.

Schiaparelli was Chanel's antithesis: Chanel was restrained while Schiaparelli was flamboyant. Her clothes featured wild prints and unusual shapes— her collaborations with Salvador Dalí, like the "Lobster Dress" and the "Shoe Hat," are particularly well known (see "Fashion and Art"). Her creativity and daring was nothing short of brilliant. She pushed fashion toward the whimsical and the weird.

Couture went through a very dark period during World War II. Many designers fled France (including Schiaparelli); Chanel stayed, and was later accused of collaborating with the Nazis (see "Fashion Ethics"). The Nazis wanted to move the fashion business to Vienna and Berlin, and it was only through the efforts of Lucien Lelong, then head of the Chambre syndicale de la haute couture, that it remained in Paris. Even so, only twenty couture houses stayed open during the occupation. In a bid to rebuild the industry, Lelong recruited two up-and-coming designers, Pierre Balmain and Christian Dior, and put them in a studio together in 1941. After the war, Lelong's two acolytes went into business on their own. Balmain set up his own couture shop almost immediately, and was the darling of the fashion press by 1946. But Dior made a far bigger splash. His couture house opened in 1947, and his very first collection revolutionized the aesthetics of

right — In flowing silk organza with horsehair embroidery, Elsa Schiaparelli's "Lobster Dress" was a gloriously strange collaboration with Surrealist artist Salvador Dalí of 1937.

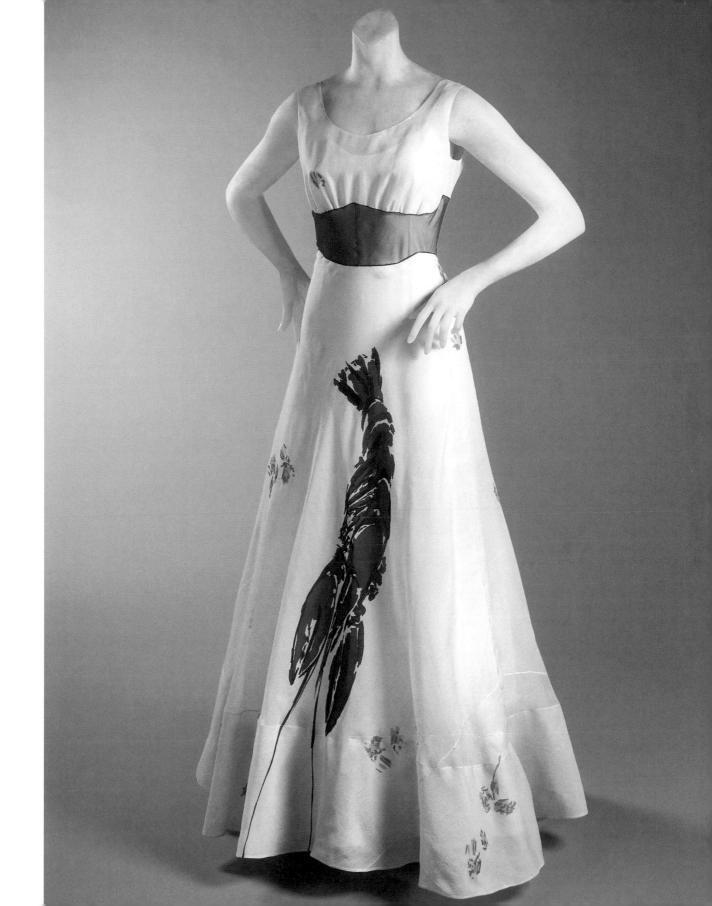

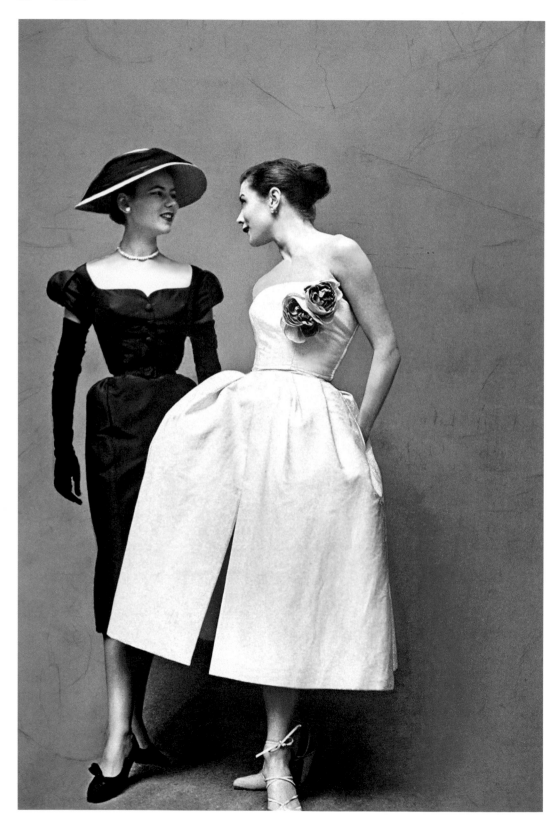

the time. Practicality went out the window; Dior's New Look (as it was later dubbed by Carmel Snow) was all about ultrafeminine curves, crisp tailoring, full skirts, and an accentuated hip and bust. It was an utter rejection of wartime rationing and represented a return to the feminine ideals of the past. The couture industry's health surged in the fifties, and following the war there were 106 couture houses. But that all changed during the sixties. The postwar baby boomers were coming of age, making youthful fashions popular and demanding clothes they could afford. And of course, designers adapted, with many focusing their attentions on more accessible ready-to-wear (see "Ready-to-Wear and Mass Fashion"). By the seventies, there were only nineteen couture houses.

The seventies were a tough time for couture. It wasn't just the triumph of ready-to-wear; the bleak economic situation drove down sales in the US, formerly couture's biggest client. The industry needed to restructure in order to survive. Between 1973 and 1975 the organizations representing haute couture and ready-to-wear (the successors to the Chambre syndicale) joined forces to represent designers at a broader level in an organization called the Fédération française de la couture du prêt-à-porter des couturiers and créateurs de mode. But bigger changes were to come. In the eighties, LVMH, a French-owned luxury brand conglomerate, remade the entire structure of the fashion industry. Starting with the merger of Louis Vuitton and Moët Hennessy, LVMH went on to control a large portfolio of luxury fashion brands, including Christian Dior (purchased in 1984). Throughout the nineties, LVMH's powerful CEO Bernard Arnault bought up a wide swathe of other brands, including Dior, Givenchy, Celine, and Kenzo, making LVMH a bona fide couture empire. In the late nineties, LVMH's moves were echoed by PPR (renamed Kering in 2013), another luxury conglomerate that acquired Alexander McQueen, Gucci, Balenciaga, and other companies.

At LVMH, Arnault's moves went beyond simple restructuring. He also orchestrated some daring creative ventures, such as founding the house of Christian Lacroix. Lacroix caused a stir, but ultimately his label failed to ever turn a profit and it was sold by LVMH in 2005 (and lost funding entirely in 2009). Arnault did have an eye for talent, however, sagely appointing a young Alexander McQueen chief designer for Givenchy, where he worked from 1996 to 2001 before forming his much-loved eponymous

left — Cinched waists, full skirts, and demure hourglass figures: Dior's New Look was a return to classic feminine ideals.

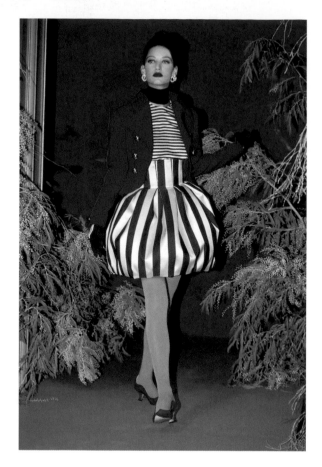

label. Around the same time, many prophesized the death of couture—until bad-boy provocateur Jean Paul Gaultier launched his first couture collection in 1997. By the early aughts the press proclaimed him a savior of the art, with collections that infused couture with lavish sexuality.

Despite the influence of conglomerates, independent couture still has a place, sometimes willfully so. Publicly traded Hermès continues to resist becoming part of LVMH, buying back shares to keep the luxury goods company within the family. New couturiers continue to spring up, too, such as Bouchra Jarrar and Alexis Mabille.

Recently, the picture has looked a little rosier for couture, though for somewhat dark reasons. During 2008's world financial crisis, much was made of the 1 percent, that wealthiest strata of society that became significantly richer during the twenty-first century. No surprise: extremely wealthy people were able to sail easily though the financial storm. So while sales of less expensive clothing declined, couture, with dresses costing in the tens to hundreds of thousands, has actually expanded. Some houses, like Armani and Valentino, have reported sales increasing by as much as 80 percent. It's hard to predict the fate of couture, but as long as wealthy people keep buying this very expensive art form, Kanye will still have something to rap about—and the rest of us will have something to envy.

above — Christian Lacroix's bubble dress wooed the women of the 1980s with its joyous, self-indulgent frivolity.

right — With their exotic sensuality and wild creativity, controversial couturier Jean Paul Gaultier's designs earned him a reputation as the savior of couture.

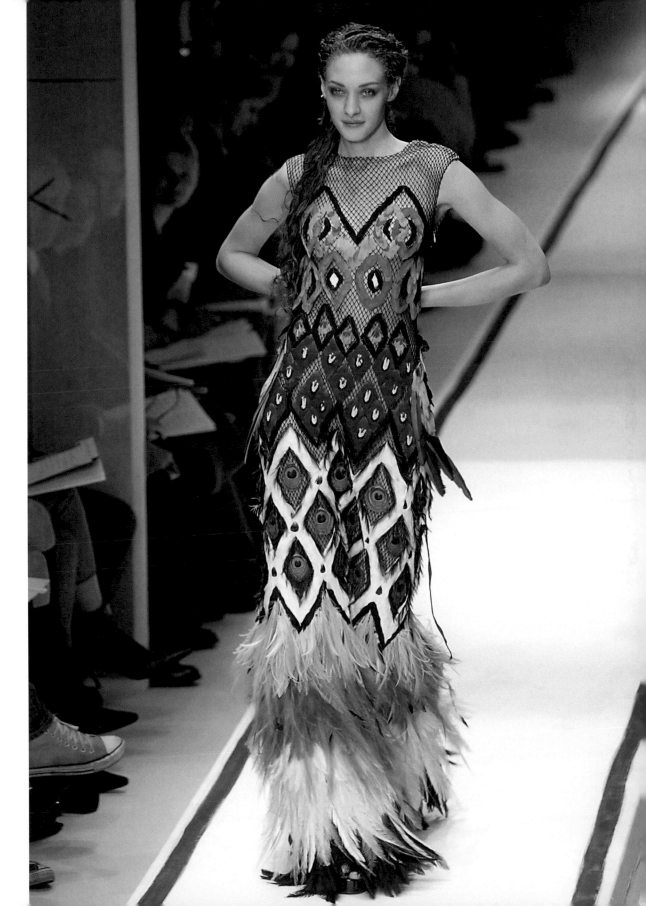

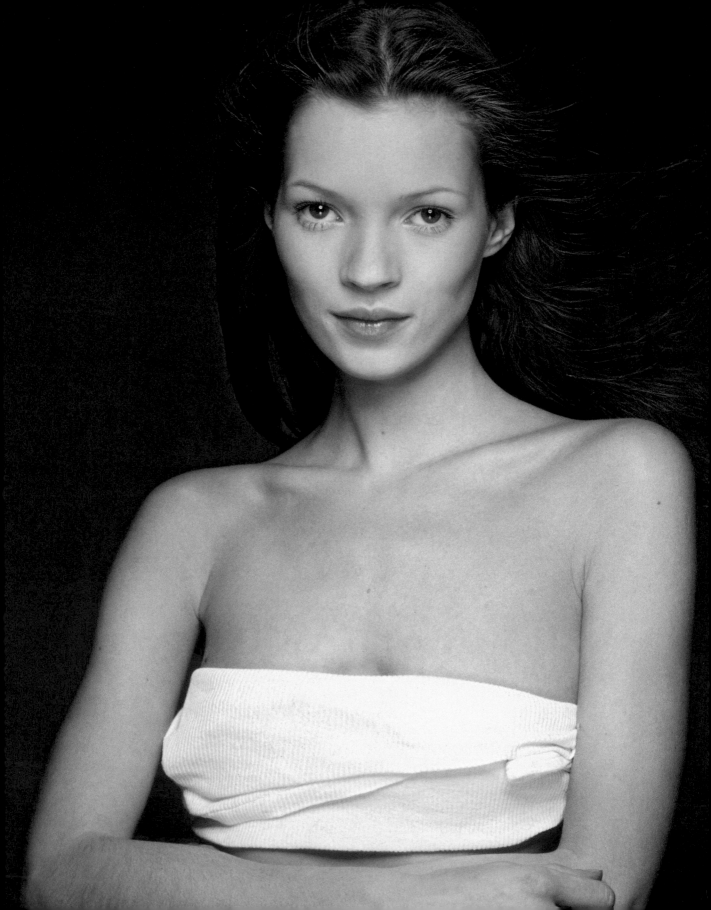

Fashion Models

Dovima, Twiggy, Naomi, Kate. When a person drops one of these names, they're talking about more than just a person; they're invoking a whole set of ideals specific to a time, whether the refined fifties, the Swinging Sixties, or the self-indulgent nineties. Nobody evokes the zeitgeist quite like models, those particularly beautiful humans chosen to represent the realities and dreams of a generation through image.

Models and couture were born at the same time, and at the hand of the same person: Charles Frederick

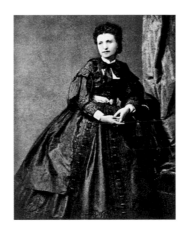

Worth, the pioneer of haute couture (see "Couture"). The English-born, Paris-based fashion designer met his future wife, Marie Vernet, when she was a shawl model. After they married they set up shop together in 1858. He designed clothing; she modeled it. This was an uncommon practice at the time—most designers used wood or straw mannequins, and when live models came into the picture, they were also called mannequins. Marie Vernet was the first in-house mannequin, modeling designs in the salon for private clients until the 1870s. After her, models typically worked in-house for a particular designer, a practice that lasted for several decades. It was a poorly paid profession, and considered fairly tawdry.

Though mannequins typically worked in-house, it wasn't long before something resembling fashion shows appeared: "mannequin parades." The first of these was launched in the 1890s by the London fashion designer Lucile (Lady Duff Gordon). She trained her models in deportment and gave them all audacious stage names—Hebe, Gamela, and Dolores. They broke ground by modeling clothing for audiences and posing dramatically, putting

left — With her unusual, gamine beauty and fearless attitude, Kate Moss (photographed here in 1995 by Terry O'Neill) forged a chameleonic, brazenly successful modeling career that's made her a true icon.

above — As the first model, Marie Vernet Worth paved the way for couture's success, winning her husband Charles Frederick Worth's creations a place in the wardrobes of powerful women such as Eugénie de Montijo, Napoleon's wife.

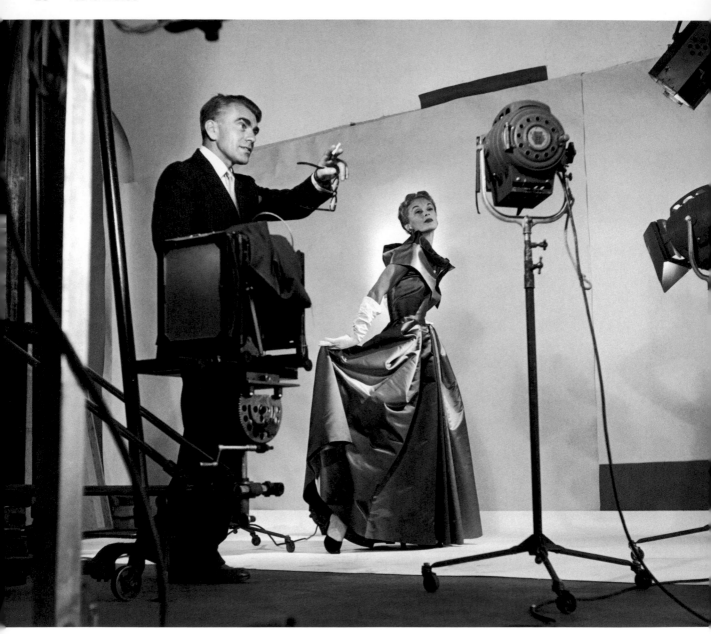

on the kind of show we take for granted in runway models today.

The advent of photography brought a new specialization to modeling, as camera-friendly beauty became marketable. There were still house models, for whom a charismatic personality for charming clients was a bigger asset than a pretty face, and photographic modeling, which was all about aesthetics, became a separate vocation. The first photographic models in the early twentieth century weren't professional models, but rather women recognizable for their stylish reputations, usually actresses or society women, often photographed by Baron de Meyer (see "Fashion Photography"). But it quickly became clear that status meant little in a photograph, opening the doors to models from all walks of life.

left — Some call Lisa Fonssagrives the first supermodel, and her icy Nordic glamour and dramatic curves were ideal for modeling Dior's New Look. In this photo from 1949, Horst P. Horst prepares to shoot the legendary beauty.

In the 1920s, the first photographic model to achieve some recognition was Marion Morehouse, a favorite of that era's premier fashion photographer, Edward Steichen. With her slender, boyish frame and her sleek hairstyles, Morehouse captured the rebellious flapper attitude in Steichen's modernist shots.
But the first model with palpable celebrity (some call her the first supermodel) was Lisa Fonssagrives. Born in Sweden, Fonssagrives had an hourglass figure and an imperious beauty that translated well to the pages of magazines. She began modeling in 1936 for photographers like Horst P. Horst, but she was at the height of her career at the same time as Dior's New Look changed the reigning aesthetic. The New Look (so named by the editor-in-chief of *Harper's Bazaar*, Carmel Snow) used structured garments to mold the body into an ultrafeminine silhouette with accentuated bust and hips. Fonssagrives possessed both the curvaceous body and the haughty attitude to really make the New Look work, and her collaborations with photographer Irving Penn (whom she married in 1950) are legendary.
Other contemporaries of Fonssagrives included Dovima, an exotic beauty who famously modeled for Richard Avedon ("Dovima with the Elephants" being a particularly well-known shot), Dorian Leigh, and Suzy Parker. Leigh and Parker were actually

sisters, with Leigh becoming famous first; her father wouldn't let her use the family name because he thought modeling, with its bad reputation, might tarnish it. Leigh, notably, fought for and opened Paris's first modeling agency in the fifties (the first one in the United States was founded decades earlier by John Powers, in 1923).
The Parker sisters may have both been models, but physically, they were quite different: Leigh stood under five foot five, while Parker was five foot ten. At the time, Parker was considered too tall to be a model, but she persisted, and alongside Fonssagrives often receives the "first supermodel" designation. Her lanky frame was a precursor to the tall, leggy look of models from the sixties to today.
In the sixties, the division between house models and photographic models weakened, meaning that models could work across the disciplines. But more importantly, the youth-centered cultural revolution turned aesthetics on their head (see "Fashion Subcultures"). Out were the hourglass curves of the New Look, and in were fresh, young, street-influenced styles. Ready-to-wear clothes gained traction over couture, and catwalk shows such as Mary Quant's emphasized flair and drama. Jean Shrimpton modeled through this transition; her snub-nosed, doe-eyed appearance was at once

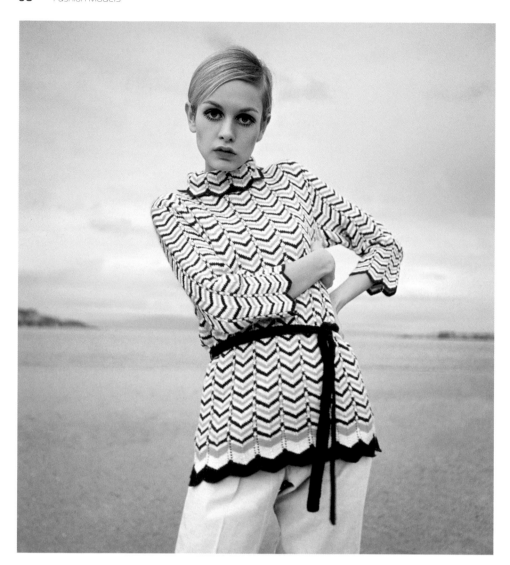

youthful but still classically pretty. But the real sea change came with one of the twentieth century's most influential models, Twiggy.

London-born Lesley Lawson received the nickname "Twiggy" for her famously boyish, slender frame. She was only sixteen when she started modeling, and her childish looks made clear youth's new supremacy, and confirmed the ascent of androgynous beauty. Twiggy experienced worldwide fame, becoming such an icon of the sixties that her photo was sent into space in a time capsule.

The antiestablishment aesthetic revolution of the six-ties also paved the way for more diversity in models. China Machado, a gorgeous part-Portuguese, part-Chinese model, made waves as the first non-Caucasian to appear in a fashion magazine (she landed a 1958 spread in *Harper's Bazaar*, at Richard Avedon's insistence, and later worked as a fashion editor for the magazine). Meanwhile, Donyale Luna was the first black model to grace the cover of British *Vogue* in 1966 (American *Vogue* didn't see its first black cover model until 1977, with Beverly Johnson). Around the same time, Japanese model Hiroko Matsumoto became well known modeling for Pierre Cardin. Models like these paved the way for the success of others, like the Somali beauty

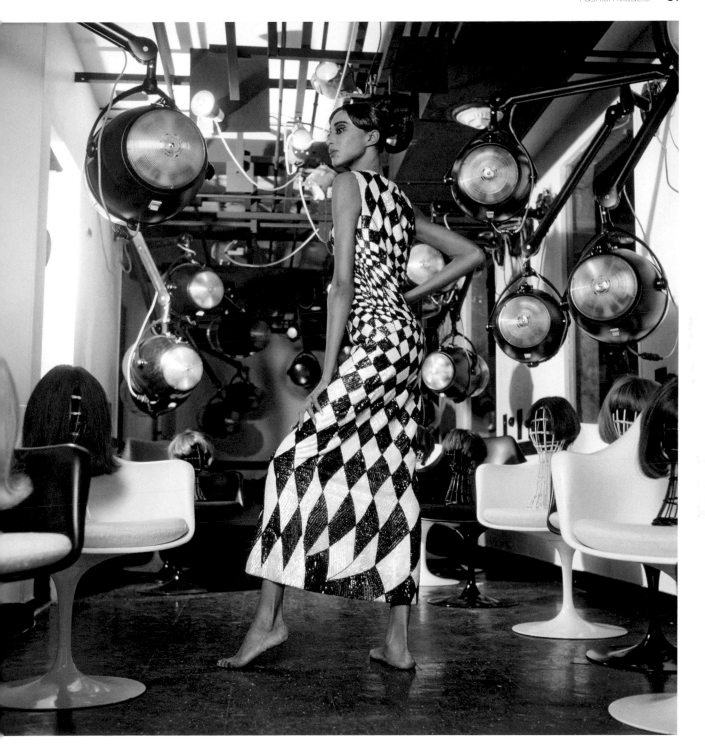

above — Finally, a little diversity: Detroit-born Donyale Luna was the first black cover girl, appearing on British *Vogue* in 1966 (shot here in the same year by Patrice Habans).

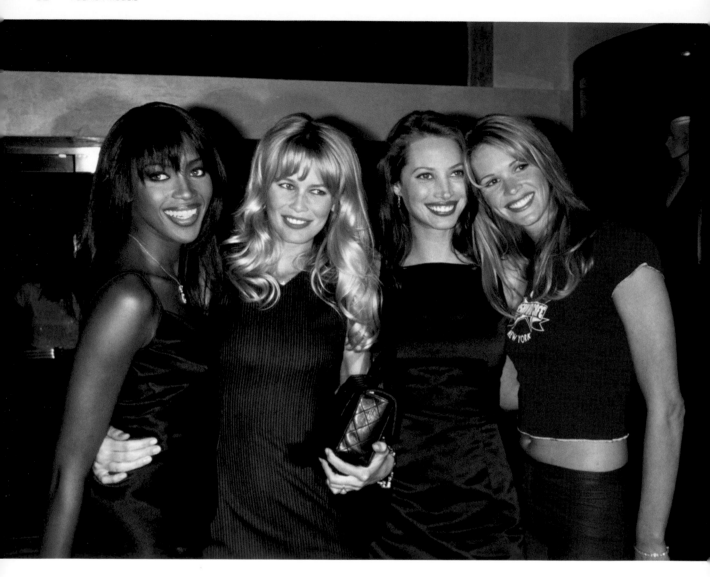

above — Global fashion empires needed powerful ambassadors, and awe-inspiringly famous supermodels like Naomi, Claudia, Christy, and Elle (shown here in 1995) were the result.

Iman, who rose to great fame in the following decades.

By the seventies, the cultural furor that marked the previous decade was over, and fashion refocused on working women and practical choices (see "Feminism and Fashion"). There was no better model to embody those ideals than the naturally quirky Lauren Hutton. Gap-toothed and lanky, she had a down-to-earth look that women related to. Hutton's relatability only enhanced her power, and she scored an exclusive cosmetics contract with Revlon worth $500,000—groundbreaking at the time. Margaux Hemingway followed suit the next year with a $1 million contract with Fabergé. These high-paying contracts helped generate fame for the two models. But even the level of fame achieved by Hutton and Hemingway was no match for what came next: the supermodels. Though the term was tossed around as early as the 1940s, "supermodel" came to refer to a particular group of highly paid models from the mid-eighties and early nineties: Christy Turlington, Naomi Campbell, Stephanie Seymour, Linda Evangelista, Tatjana Patitz, and later Cindy Crawford and Claudia Schiffer.

There were a few factors that contributed to the dramatic rise of the supermodels. One was the general culture of excess in the eighties that supported the celebration of conspicuous consumption and obvious wealth. Another was the tendency of some photographers (notably Steven Meisel) to shoot with the same models over and over again, making them familiar faces. But most important was the conglomeration of fashion labels in the eighties—many formerly independent brands were purchased by large multinationals like LVMH and PPR (for more on the mergers, see "Couture"). These huge companies were more than willing to invest in big-budget advertising campaigns to reach a worldwide audience and expand their market around the globe. A side effect of these ad campaigns was the unprecedented level of exposure they gave the models, making them as famous as movie stars.

By the mid-nineties, the stock market had crashed and the excesses of the eighties were passé—and the supermodels began their decline. Grunge aesthetics, anti-mainstream sentiment, and "heroin chic" became the vogue. This atmosphere of disaffection was the perfect storm that launched the next big modeling sensation: Kate Moss. Standing only five foot six with an off-kilter beauty, a sullen attitude, and a waifish frame that would inspire controversy about whether she was a healthy role model, she was everything that the tall, buxom supermodels were not. At the same time as Kate was on the ascent, celebrities were also beginning to take the place of models: magazine editors like Anna Wintour started to feature them on covers and in fashion spreads, to much commercial success (see "Celebrity Fashion").

Some models still get billed as supermodels (Heidi Klum and Gisele Bündchen are of particular note), but overall, modeling in the twenty-first century has become more diverse, with more opportunities for models with unusual looks or figures that haven't traditionally been embraced by fashion. One example is plus-size modeling. Once operating as a fringe industry, plus-size models have seen mainstream exposure: notable are Kate Dillon, who was the first plus-sized model to appear in American *Vogue*, in 2001, and Crystal Renn, who appeared in John Galliano's 2006 catwalk show to great acclaim. (Renn later lost a great deal of weight, to much controversy.) Older models gained popularity, too; China Machado again made headlines when IMG signed her to their roster in 2011, making her the oldest signed model at age eighty-one.

The gay, lesbian, and transgender rights movement gained major ground in the new millennium, so it's no surprise that gender issues have become visible in modeling. One gender-bending model of particular note is Andrej Pejić, a Bosnian-Australian male whose delicate, feminine beauty allows him to model in women's fashion shows (Pejić originally gained notoriety for walking in Jean Paul Gaultier's Spring 2011 catwalk shows for women). Around the same time, Lea T, a transgendered male-to-female model, made waves as Givenchy's muse and appeared in the pages of magazines like Paris *Vogue*. And then, in late 2012, French model Casey Legler signed with Ford Models as a male model—the first woman to do so.

Today's models are a world away from Marie Vernet Worth—and that's a good thing, since the world is a far different place than it was in 1858. And you can place a safe bet that come next century the models will capture the strange beauty of the future, something unknowable to us now, but by then, à la mode.

right — He makes a beautiful bride: gender-bending model Andrej Pejić walks in Jean Paul Gaultier's 2011 show, bringing androgyny to the catwalk in an era of progress for LGBT rights.

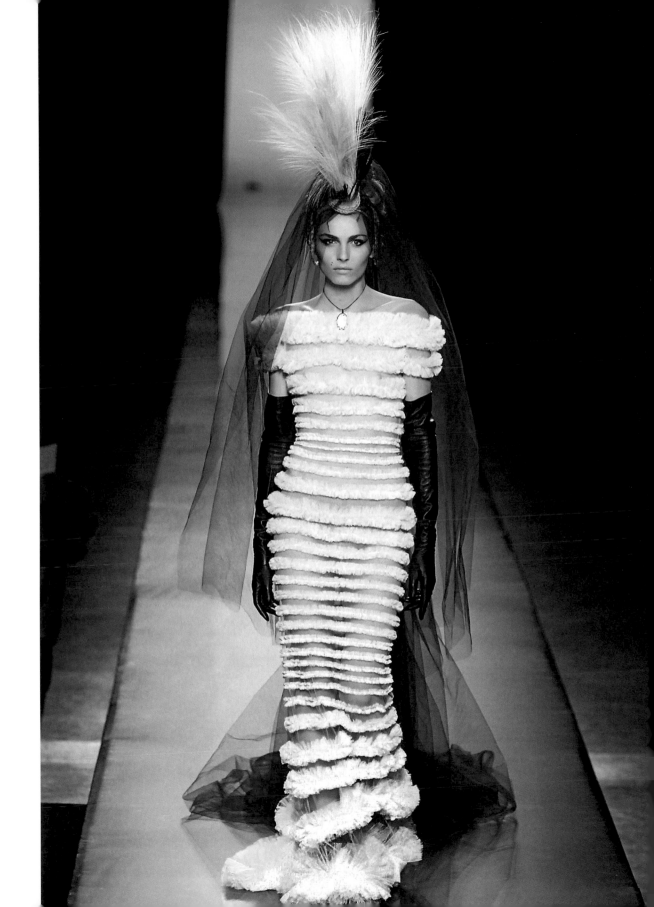

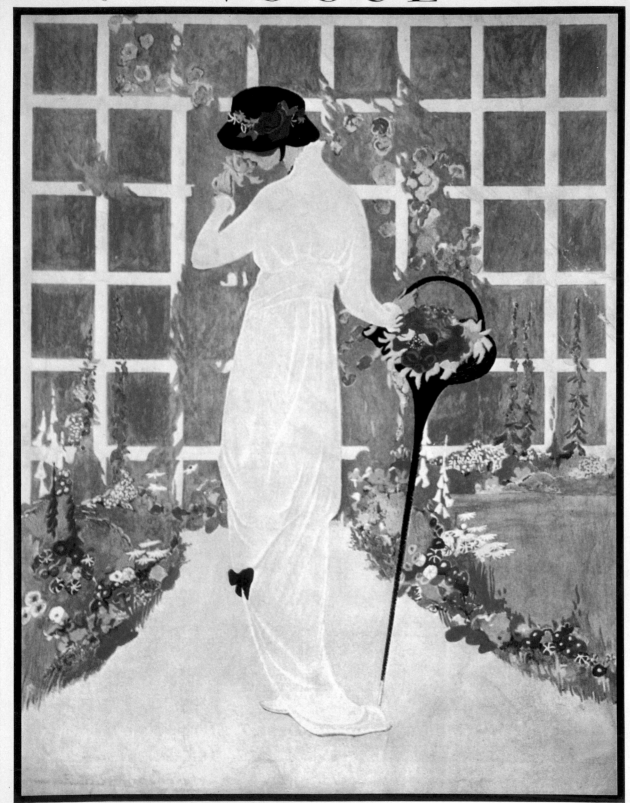

Fashion Magazines

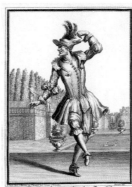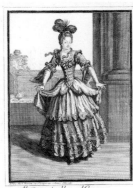

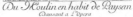

I n 2008, "Magazines are dead!" was as much a catchphrase as a prophesy by internet naysayers. The spectacular stock market crash had caused shell-shocked advertisers to pull ads, and magazines were suffering. But by 2012, *Vogue*, fashion's bible, weighed in at 916 pages—its biggest issue ever. And this despite stiff competition from fashion blogs on the internet. It turns out that fashion in print really hasn't gone out of style after all.

Fashion magazines haven't been around as long as print (which appeared in the fifteenth century), but their existence runs parallel to that of fashionable society. The beginnings of fashion magazines appeared in France during the reign of the style-obsessed Sun King, Louis XIV (see "Royal Fashion").

left — Launched in 1892, *Vogue* has been a bible of fashion for over one hundred years; this issue from 1913 shows off the magazine's early illustrative cover style.

above— The *Mercure Galant*, a French literary arts magazine from the seventeenth century, was the first to showcase fashion in its pages—these two fashion plates show off some truly vintage styles for upper-class men and women.

The first magazine to feature fashion was the *Mercure Galant*, a French gazette of the literary arts and society launched in 1672 by playwright Molière's rival Jean Donneau de Visé. De Visé didn't have much success as a playwright, but he did make his mark with the *Mercure*. A tastemaking publication of the elite, it went beyond arts journalism to include regular coverage of contemporary style. Fashions were represented by printed engravings, similar to the single-sheet fashion plates popular at the time. The *Mercure* was a financial success, and continued regular fashion coverage up until 1679 (around which time, importantly, it covered fashionable society's evasion of the sumptuary laws, the ordinances banning people from dressing outside their class). Though it has dropped fashion coverage, the *Mercure*, called since 1972 *Mercure de France*, continues to be an influential voice in the arts today.

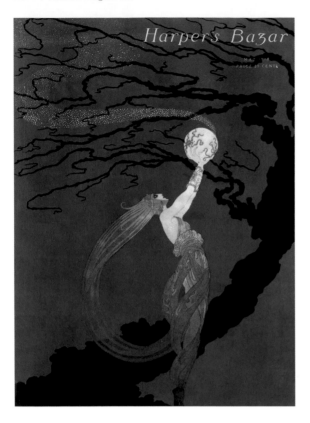

Despite these earlier French efforts, the first dedicated fashion magazines didn't appear for another two centuries. In 1867, *Harper's Bazar* (it got the second *a* in 1929) was launched as a weekly newspaper format publication, edited by Mary Louise Booth. Its tagline was "a repository of fashion, pleasure, and instruction." Its chief rival, *Vogue*, launched in 1892, also a weekly. Initially, both publications were society magazines detailing the lives of the upper classes, featuring illustrations of mostly European fashions, as well as information on where to buy them.

But the pivotal moment came in 1909, when Condé Montrose Nast, a lawyer turned advertising salesman, bought *Vogue* and transformed it into a bona fide fashion magazine. Coming from an advertising background, Nast had a keen understanding of niche markets, and saw the growing body of female consumers for what they were: a huge opportunity. When he bought *Vogue*, he pushed the content heavily toward fashion, and changed it to a biweekly. Soon after, in 1913, William Randolph Hearst bought *Harper's*, repositioning it as *Vogue*'s

direct competitor. The rivalry lasted for years, and the two men founded what were to become America's biggest magazine publishers, Condé Nast and Hearst Publications.

There were some small but noteworthy experiments in fashion magazines during that era as well. From 1912 through 1925, Condé Nast published a magazine called *La Gazette du Bon Ton*. A super high-end affair, it was a subscriber-only publication that, today, would cost in the hundreds of dollars per year. Interestingly, the magazine maintained contracts with the major couture houses of the time so that illustrations of their designs (often done by the major Art Deco illustrators) would appear exclusively in *Bon Ton*.

above — *Harper's Bazaar* began life as a society magazine, later becoming one of the first dedicated fashion magazines, alongside *Vogue*. This issue from 1918 features a cover design by the Russian artist Erté.

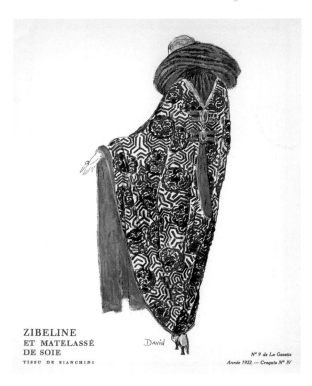

ZIBELINE
ET MATELASSÉ
DE SOIE
TISSU DE BIANCHINI

N° 9 de La Gazette
Année 1922. — Croquis N° IV

After the invention of photography, illustration in fashion magazines began a slow fade. The first fashion photographs in a magazine appeared in *La Mode Pratique* in 1892 (though Edward Steichen's images of Paul Poiret gowns in *Art & Décoration* in 1911 often claim first-ran status). From that point on, the development of fashion magazines and fashion photography were tightly intertwined (see "Fashion Photography").

Fashion magazines experienced a major creative evolution in the 1940s, mostly led by a brilliantly creative triumvirate of people at *Harper's Bazaar*: editor Carmel Snow, art director Alexey Brodovitch, and fashion editor Diana Vreeland. Snow was known for sniffing out talent, and Brodovitch and Vreeland were two examples of her ability to do so.

Brodovitch, in particular, radically changed the look of fashion magazines. A Russian-born designer who fled to Paris during the Bolshevik Revolution, Brodovitch brought his experience with the European avant-garde to the magazine's pages. He used his connections to get artists like Marc Chagall, Jean Cocteau, and Man Ray to contribute, exposing mainstream American magazine audiences to edgy European artists. Most of all he is known for introducing movement to layouts through cinematic arrangement of fanned images and text that almost seemed to dance across the page through plenty of white space.

And then there was Diana Vreeland, a figure so iconic among fashion editors that she was immortalized as the character Maggie Prescott in the film *Funny Face*. Carmel Snow discovered her dancing in a white Chanel dress at the St. Regis Hotel, and instantly saw her as an essential addition to the *Bazaar* team. While at *Harper's* she penned her unforgettable fashion advice column "Why Don't You?," in which she recommended things that

above — Subscriber-only *La Gazette du Bon Ton* (pictured here from 1922) thrived on exclusivity, with unique fashion illustrations and a price tag affordable for only the privileged.

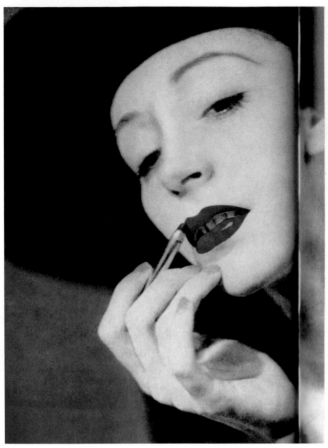

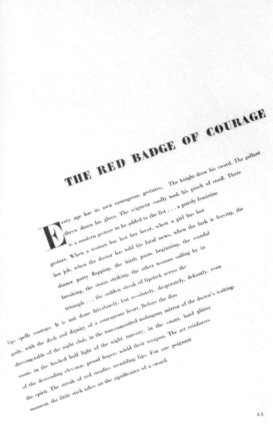

ranged from the sublime to the bizarre, like "Why don't you... wash your blond child's hair in dead champagne, as they do in France?" It was whimsical to say the least.

When Carmel Snow left *Harper's* in 1958, Vreeland pinned her hopes on the position of editor in chief. When she didn't get the job, she waited three years and then seized the opportunity to edit *Vogue* (considered a betrayal, at the time). It was a fateful move: during her time at *Vogue*, Vreeland changed the magazine completely, making it the preeminent fashion title of the times almost by sheer force of her personality. Vreeland's tenure at *Vogue* coincided with the youth revolution of the sixties, and she managed to transfer its free-spirited ideology to the magazine's pages. She favored models with an unusual beauty, like Veruschka and Cher—really, she was

the first to exploit the idea of the model as personality. She also took photography out of the studio and into exotic locales, traveling around the world for fashion shoots in far-flung places.

Working with her was art director Alexander Liberman. Like Brodovitch, Liberman was a Russian émigré who used his European art connections to the magazine's advantage—including scooping Salvador Dalí to illustrate the occasional cover. Coming from the newsmagazine *Vu*, Liberman took a different approach than Brodovitch, favoring crowded pages, messy layouts, and little white space. Notably, he also emphasized text on the magazine's cover describing what a reader would find inside—the origin of the noisy cover lines on contemporary magazines.

In 1971, *Vogue*'s management decided the magazine should be more grounded, less glamorous, and

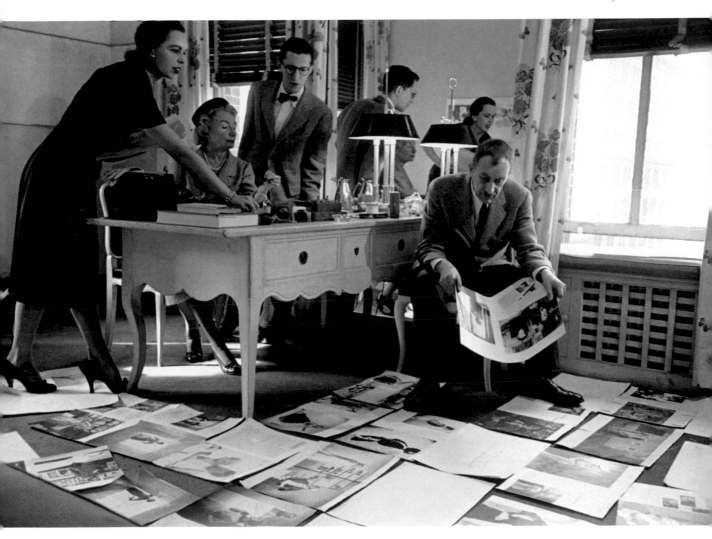

left — Perhaps the most famous magazine art director of all
time, Alexey Brodovitch brought motion and white space to
the page, along with a raft of art-world contacts. This *Harper's
Bazaar* layout from 1937 features photography by Man Ray
and a radical layout by Brodovitch.

above — Artistic alchemy: Carmel Snow led *Harper's Bazaar*
through a period of creative ferment; she's shown here examin-
ing the magazine's layout with art director Alexey Brodovitch
in 1952.

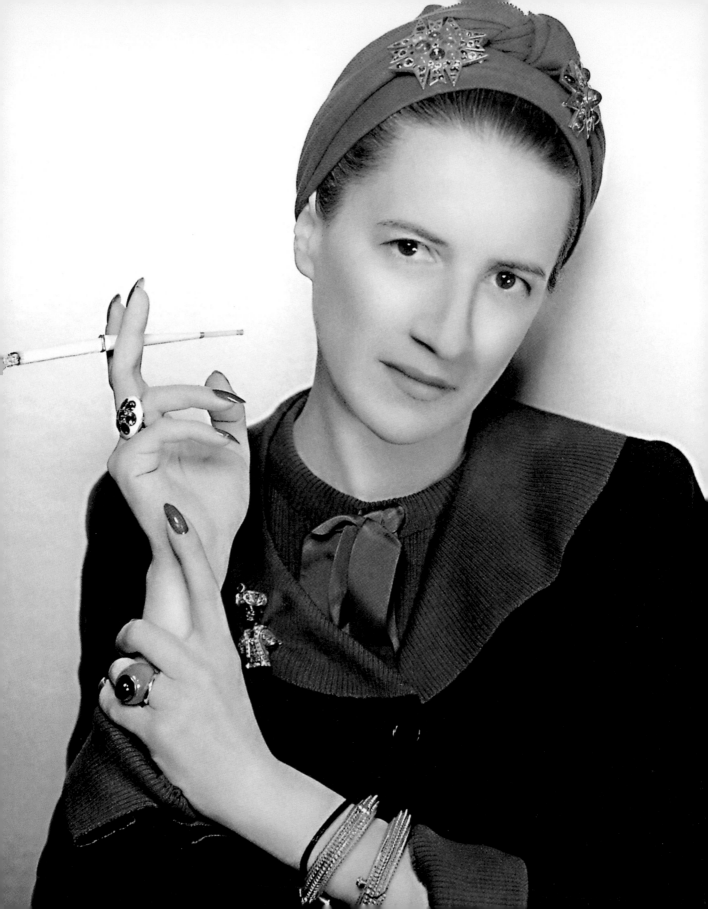

Diana Vreeland was dismissed. After she left, *Vogue* focused more on working women and lifestyle under editor Grace Mirabella (who literally took Vreeland's red-walled and leopard-skin-carpeted office and painted it beige). But then, in 1988, the ferociously bob-haired Anna Wintour took over and reinvigorated *Vogue* with a sense of style. Coming from a family of journalists, she was a savvy businesswoman, and turned the magazine into a fashion powerhouse. She championed a high/low style of dressing that incorporated couture and cheaper ready-to-wear, while her fashion shoots returned to the big-picture, story-based shoots favored by Vreeland rather than the studio-shot photos Mirabella had employed. Her other big move was putting celebrities on the cover of the magazine (see "Celebrity Fashion"), a tactic that broadened the magazine's popular appeal and amped up newsstand sales.

left — A brilliant iconoclast, Diana Vreeland did things her own way, bringing boundless creativity to her periods at *Harper's Bazaar* and *Vogue*.

Like Carmel Snow, Wintour surrounded herself with talent, hiring André Leon Talley as editor at large and Grace Coddington as creative director. The fiery-maned Coddington herself became a fashion icon when the documentary *The September Issue* hit the screens in 2009, a movie that revealed her as the creative genius behind the romantic fashion story-books *Vogue* was famous for.

At the same time as *Vogue* dominated the newsstands, independent fashion magazines catering to more edgy tastes proliferated, such as *The Face* (founded in 1980 by Nick Logan), *i-D* (founded in 1980 by Terry Jones), *Dazed & Confused* (founded in 1992 by Jefferson Hack and Rankin), and *Purple* (founded in 1992 by Elein Fleiss and Olivier Zahm). One particularly notable title from this time was *Visionaire* (1991), a multi-format limited edition fashion and art publication. Still running today, it caters to a very niche audience willing to shell out hundreds, sometimes thousands of dollars for unique collector's editions. One of the most talked about was issue number 18, which came in a custom-designed Louis Vuitton portfolio. *Visionaire* is proof that ultra-high end can absolutely work, particularly in a limited run.

In the wake of 2008's financial crisis, most magazines shrank, and many went under.

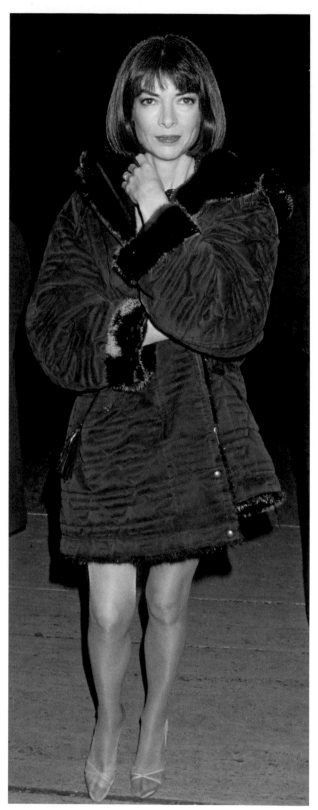

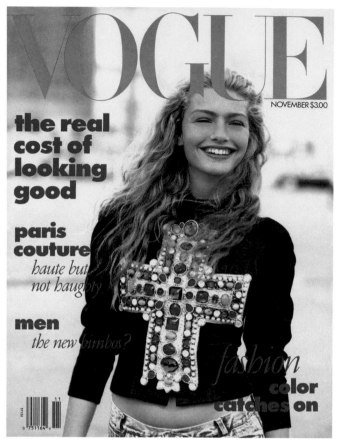

above — *Vogue*'s first cover under Anna Wintour's leadership in 1988 exemplified high/low dressing, with the casual pairing of a Christian Lacroix couture jacket with Guess jeans.

left — Fiercely businesslike, Anna Wintour (shown here in 1991) knew how to make fashion work, transforming *Vogue* into the reader-friendly, celebrity-fronted success story that it is today.

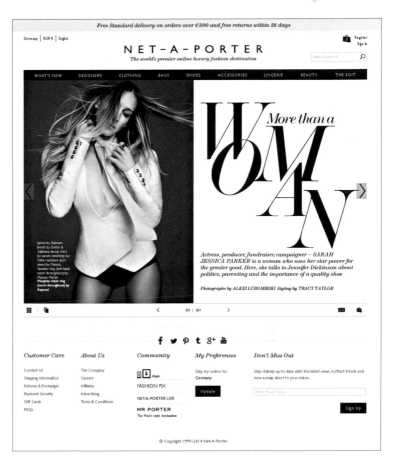

In an environment of smaller budgets and online competition, brands themselves took the plunge into magazine publishing. Rather than placing ads in multiple magazines, they could make their own and control the voice, image, and styling to all be consistent with their brand. Many branded magazines cover things outside of fashion, and aim for the authenticity and relative editorial freedom allowed by the major magazines (save for the clothes the models wear, usually). Branded magazines can

above — With ample white space, beautiful photographs, and playful typography, web magazines often pay homage to their print lineage, as seen in this spread from Net-a-Porter's online magazine *The Edit*.

afford to pay editors well—and so they pulled talent from some major titles in a quick, noticeable manner. For example: Lucy Yeomans, editor in chief of *Harper's Bazaar* UK left her position for a job at online luxury retailer Net-a-Porter's magazine, while *Marie Claire's* Taylor Tomasi Hill moved to Moda Operandi; others continue to follow suit. And yet, *Vogue* grows fatter by the year. Despite the proliferation of blogs and branded online publications, print fashion magazines continue to thrive; perhaps it's because there is something particularly beautiful about photography in print. Meanwhile, online publications strive to mimic the style and tone of print publications, using editorial layouts that look much like what you'd see on a printed page—echoes of Alexey Brodovitch in the digital world. It may not be the golden age of print anymore, but magazines, it seems, still rule fashion.

Fashion Photography

There is a scene in Michelangelo Antonioni's 1966 film *Blow-Up* in which a photographer kneels over a writhing model (played by Veruschka), snapping frantically as she undulates erotically. These days, the scene plays like a cliché—a fashion photographer pointing a camera at a lissome model is as much a stock image as a painter at an easel before a Rubenesque nude. And that's because photography has defined fashion for more than a century, acquainting us with its own particular artistry. Though photographs of people in stylish clothes have existed since photography began in 1839, true fashion photography didn't bloom until the invention of halftone printing allowed the mass reproduction of images (see "Fashion Magazines"). The first fashion photographs popped up in France in 1881, in pattern books; the first printed fashion photographs appeared in 1892 in a French magazine called *La Mode Pratique*. But in many history books, the founder of fashion photography is cited as Edward Steichen, for his 1911 photos of Paul Poiret dresses in *Art & Décoration*—probably because, in his autobiography, he claimed they were "probably the first serious fashion photographs ever made." Whether he was making a snide comment on the seriousness of previous fashion photographs is unclear. After Steichen's photos in 1911, he vanished from fashion photography until 1923. In the interim, fashion's most prominent photographer was Baron de Meyer, whose romantic backlit shots featuring soft focus, flowers, and ornamentation were all about creating a mood. He was the staff photographer for Condé Nast until 1923, by which point his photographic style was so imitated that it became passé. He was replaced by none other than Edward Steichen, who threw out all the backlighting and bric-a-brac in favor of clean, decisive modernism, with flapper models shot in plain settings. Fashion photography lost its posed formality in 1933, when Hungarian photographer Martin Munkácsi burst onto the scene. Before being hired by Carmel Snow at *Harper's Bazaar*, Munkácsi was a sports photographer, which meant he shot fashion the way he would sports: on the move. His photography had a documentary feel, capturing women in the moment, often outdoors, very much alive. His photos forever changed fashion photography, turning it into something altogether more vital.

right — Woman in motion: Martin Munkácsi's photographs for *Harper's Bazaar* (like this one from 1933) brimmed with athletic vitality.

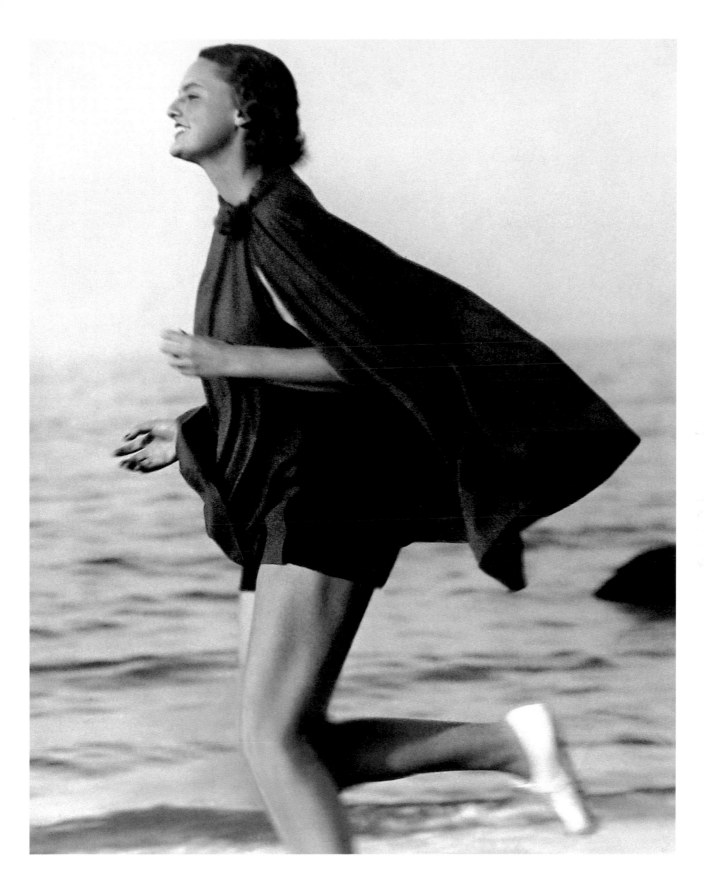

Things got a little weirder in the thirties, when Surrealism, already very much established in art, crept into photography. Its biggest proponent was Man Ray, who began working for *Harper's Bazaar* at Alexey Brodovitch's request. Fashion wasn't the main event for Man Ray, so he didn't have the same expectations as others for how clothes should appear in photos. He played with darkroom effects like distortion and solarization, which reversed the tones in a photo in an otherworldly manner. The thirties also saw an important technical innovation: color photography, with *Vogue* getting its first color cover from Edward Steichen in 1932.

In terms of overall popularity and influence, the most important fashion photographer of the era was Cecil Beaton. Beaton was fond of using detailed rococo backdrops for his shoots—hints of his involvement with costume and set design. His critical perspective on the models and celebrities he photographed was infamous; his attitude was so harsh that Jean Cocteau gave him the nickname "Malice in Wonderland." But at the same time, he did whatever it took to flatter his subjects, narrowing their waistlines and highlighting their best features with photo editing. He was also the first to contrast glamour with industrial decay, posing a group of models in front of a construction site near the Champs-Élysées in 1937. This sort of juxtaposition has been echoed, repeatedly, in fashion photography up to the present day.

Fashion photography ground to a bit of a standstill during World War II. It was considered frivolous, not to mention that fashion itself had taken a far more utilitarian direction during this time of scarce resources and rationing. But the postwar era was a hot time for fashion photography in the United States, when two of the century's biggest photographers came onto the scene: Irving Penn and Richard Avedon.

Avedon was another product of the editorial alchemy at *Harper's Bazaar*. Like that other *Harper's* photographer, Munkácsi, Avedon's shots were characterized by models in motion. Hired in 1946 at the age of twenty-one, he was a legend soon after. His photographs from the fifties, which he called "a vacation from life," depicted vivacious girls, vigorously experiencing the giddy postwar return to normal activity. When Diana Vreeland took over *Vogue*'s

right — Surrealist artist Man Ray's photography (like "The Pulse of Fashion," shown here, of 1937) put art first, and fashion second.

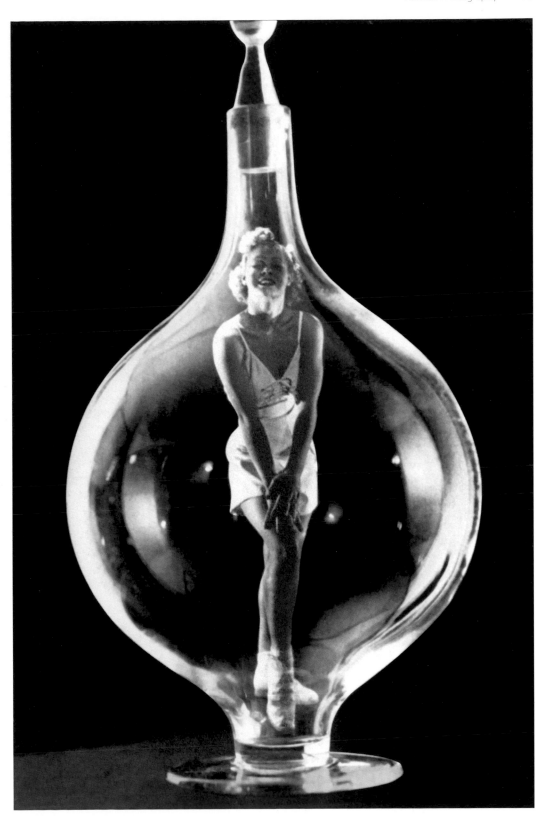

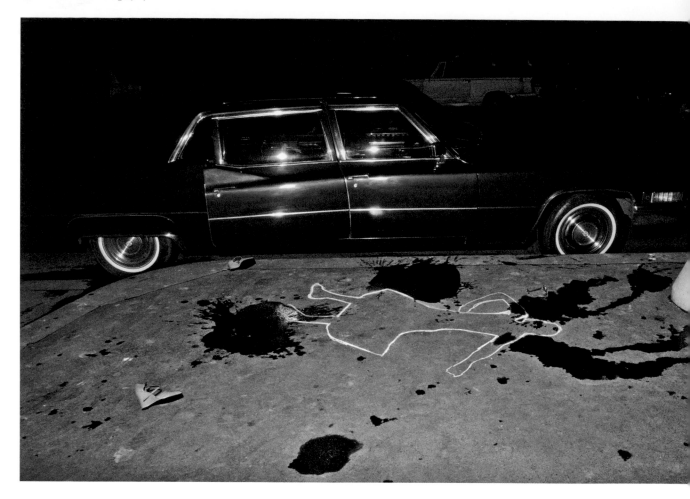

editorship in 1962, Avedon followed her, shooting almost every cover for the magazine until Anna Wintour took the helm.

Avedon's later work moved into the studio, typically shot against a plain white background. Still a fan of motion, his signature studio shot had models happily leaping for the camera.

Meanwhile, Irving Penn came into the spotlight while working as Alexander Liberman's creative assistant in 1942. He became known for his perfectly composed portraits and still lifes—his clearly defined photos of the Paris collections of the fifties, stripped bare of any background ornamentation or props, set him apart from other photographers of the time. Shooting for *Vogue* up until his death in 2009, his minimalist style and influence stretched for more than sixty years.

It was inevitable that the youth-fueled culture of the sixties (see "Subcultures") would make its mark on photography, and it did so in the form of bad-boy photographer David Bailey. Bailey was a member of the group of cockney photographers known as the "Terrible Three" (the other two were Brian Duffy and Terence Donovan), who drew inspiration from decidedly unrefined sources, like the poses of the mods and rockers. A notorious womanizer, Bailey's shots often had sexual overtones. Particularly charged were his photos of Jean Shrimpton, his

above — Sinister and cinematic, Guy Bourdin's photography (like this ad for Charles Jourdan shoes) captured the dark undercurrent of the 1970s.

girlfriend for four years. As the inspiration for the photographer in Antonioni's *Blow-Up*, his life is the stuff of pop-culture legend.

In a decade during which serial killers were celebrities and pornography triumphed as big business, it's no surprise that fashion photography became more transgressive. The prince of darkness in seventies fashion photography was Guy Bourdin, who worked for French *Vogue*. His work played with themes of voyeurism and violence, often with hints at a sinister plotline. His infamous ad for Charles Jourdan shoes is particularly iconic, depicting a shoe alongside an automobile accident. He inspired Deborah Turbeville, who used a similar style in American *Vogue*. Even more famous at the time was Helmut Newton, whose highly sexualized work depicted a wealthy jet set whose glamour was offset by sometimes perverse innuendoes. Newton's work progressed into the eighties, during which he skillfully captured an era known for its self-indulgence. Of particular note was his shot of Daryl Hannah in a bikini, calming a crying baby as her husband catches her with a younger lover.

The nineties brought both grunge and gazelle-like supermodels, and somehow, Steven Meisel can take credit for both. A one-time illustrator for Halston with a sweeping knowledge of high fashion, film, and the arts, Steven Meisel's images flaunt his cultural knowledge; with an eye for talent, he is also credited with kick-starting the careers of the nineties supermodels. His work embraces controversy, too: one example is Madonna's infamous book, *Sex*, which he shot. He's given heavy credit, alongside photographer Juergen Teller, for the "heroin chic" look of the nineties: pasty skin, sunken eyes, limp hair, and a gaunt frame, all paired with clothes that show it all off—a dangerous sort of beauty that then US president Bill Clinton vilified as "destructive" and "ugly." Meanwhile, Meisel's 1995 Calvin Klein campaign featuring young-looking, scantily clad teenagers was criticized as "kiddie porn," and eventually pulled.

But not all fashion photography is quite so edgy; particularly at mainstream fashion stalwart American *Vogue*, fashion photographs are often beautiful rather than shocking. And perhaps no modern fashion photographer has quite as much clout as Annie Leibovitz. A staff photographer at *Rolling Stone* in the seventies, she later moved on to work for both *Vogue* and *Vanity Fair*, becoming famous for her celebrity shots. Working alongside creative director Grace Coddington, she shoots the imaginative fashion storybooks *Vogue* has become so famous for in the new millennium. Some examples include a lush 2010 recreation of the life of Marie Antoinette in Versailles starring Kirsten Dunst, and a 2003 vision of *Alice in Wonderland* featuring model Natalia Vodianova.

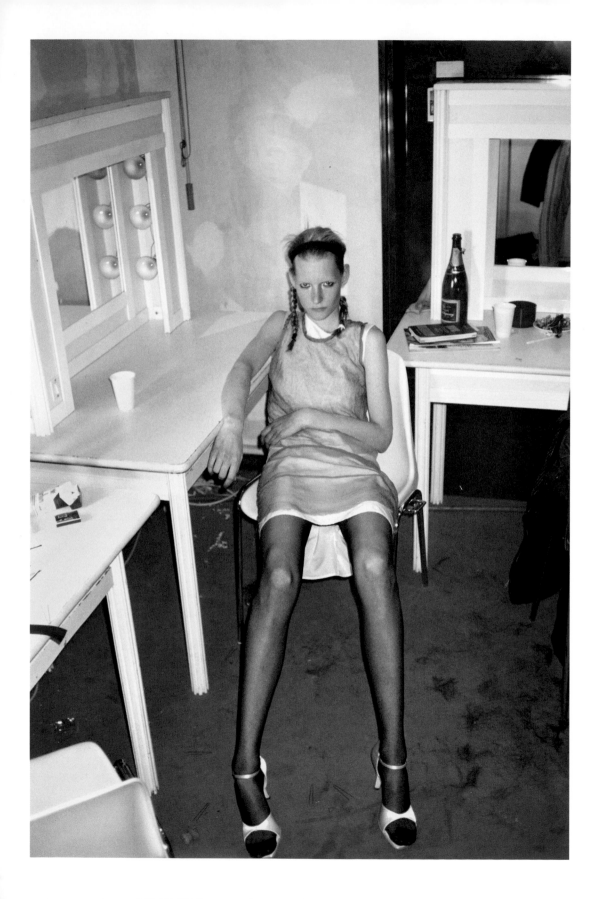

One of the more divisive issues in modern fashion photography has been the use of photo editing. Though photo editing has always existed in a basic form (often using ink and paint), digital-editing programs like Photoshop, which appeared in the nineties, paved the way for photographers to drastically alter the way people look. They'd shave off inches, and sometimes entire body parts—creating a completely unattainable beauty ideal. The debate about the ethics of photo editing came to a head in 2009, when blogs began uncovering extreme examples of digital retouching and photographer Peter Lindberg shot a series of unretouched celebrity covers for French *Elle*—images that were shocking in their naturalness. But many in the business stand up for photo editing as just another tool to help shape the fantasy of fashion.

In recent years, fashion photography has been influenced by amateur photography, an aesthetic exemplified by Terry Richardson. Richardson's lifestyle as a teen was squalid and experimental: he played music in punk bands and took part in gang bangs, experiences that made an unmistakable mark on his style. He was lucky enough to be taken under the wing of his once estranged father (sixties fashion photographer Bob Richardson), and worked his way into the world of fashion photography.

His use of point-and-shoot cameras gives his photos a spontaneous, nonprofessional, and sometimes sleazy feel, and his brightly lit studio portraits often feature full nudity and sexual acts—which, to no surprise, draw comparisons to pornography. The controversy has worked for him: Richardson's raunchy style is a big part of his fame. But by 2013 he was experiencing a media backlash due to his alleged sexual harassment of models, with repercussions like Change.org petitions advocating for brands to stop working with him.

With the internet and its multimedia immediacy, fashion photography continues to diversify, with some fashion photographers moving into video. One good example is Nick Knight's pioneering website SHOWStudio, which launched in 2000 as one of the first proponents of film in fashion. By 2013, fashion videos became so popular (and so clichéd) that they were parodied to great internet acclaim by comedian Lizzy Caplan for fashion label Vena Cava. Regardless, these fashion videos do what photography does: reflect back at us the mores of the time. They're a complementary force—if anything, reinforcing the photographic image's power to convey a message, whether still or in motion.

left — Suggesting debauched defiance, Juergen Teller's 1993 photograph of Kirsten Owen epitomizes heroin chic.

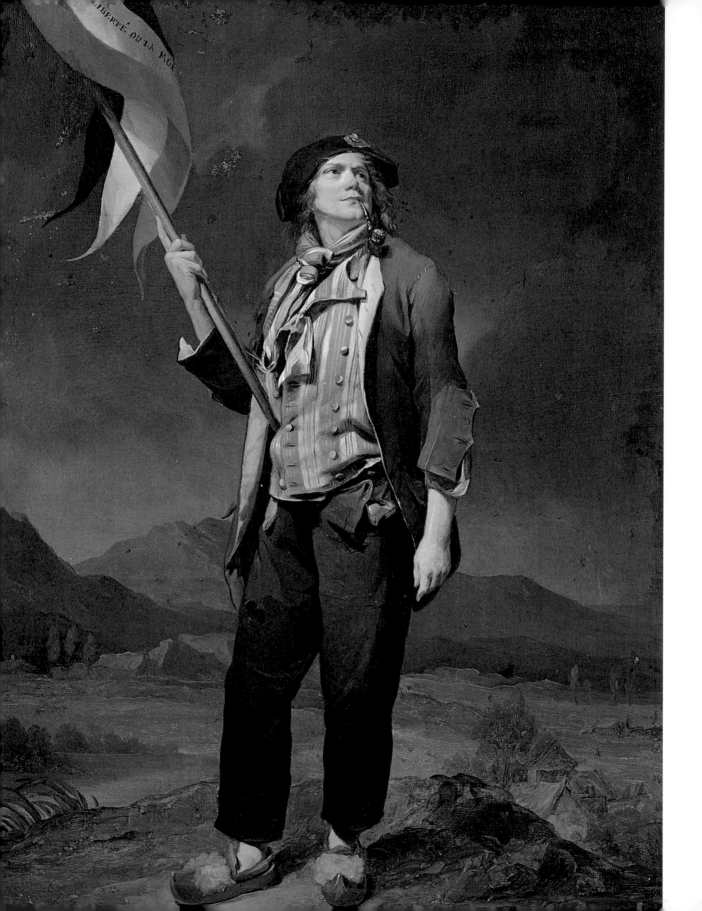

Military Fashion

Camouflage, in theory, allows a person to blend in without being seen. These days, it certainly lives up to its reputation; walking down a city street, nobody receives a second glance when wearing the stuff. It's everywhere: vintage camouflage in trendy boutiques, camo print tees in mass retailers, redesigned camouflage on the runways. Not to mention the place where it all came from: the military. Military fashion has inspired mainstream style for as long as people have donned clothes to be fashionable—and even before that. Since clothing has a real effect on battle performance, the military has long been invested in innovation in dress, and many of those ingenious developments have crept into mainstream fashion design.

One early example of the crossover between battle garb and civilian attire occurred during the Thirty Years' War, which devastated most of Europe between 1618 and 1648. Croatian mercenaries wore scarves knotted tightly around their necks, and when they came to report for military duty in Paris, the style caught on in the French capital. Originally called "à la Croate," (worn in the Croatian way), the style evolved to became a looser-tied scarf, "la cravate," the precursor to the necktie. Later, the sansculottes of the French Revolution gave greater visibility to the pantaloons worn by commoners, which wound their way into military fashions and mainstream attire and became known as trousers (see "Menswear").

The Crimean War pitted the Russian army against the allied British, French, Ottoman, and Sardinian troops between 1853 and 1856, and is sometimes cited as the first modern war. The terrible weather soldiers had to endure in the Crimea also gave us some modern fashion innovations; most significant of these is the cardigan, originally a warm knitted jacket with a wool collar. It took on the name of the Earl of Cardigan, who became famous for the Charge of the Light Brigade (given its dues in Tennyson's celebrated poem by the same name) at the Battle of Balaclava. Another weather-beating invention of the Crimean War was the balaclava itself, a knit hat with holes for eyes and mouth now best-known as an accessory for skiing and robbing banks. In 1856, outdoors outfitter Burberry was founded by Thomas Burberry; half a century later, the company became known for one of menswear's most iconic wardrobe pieces, the trench coat. (Aquascutum also

left — There was a time when wearing pants was revolutionary; shown here is a sansculotte from the French Revolution, clad in the trousers of the working class.

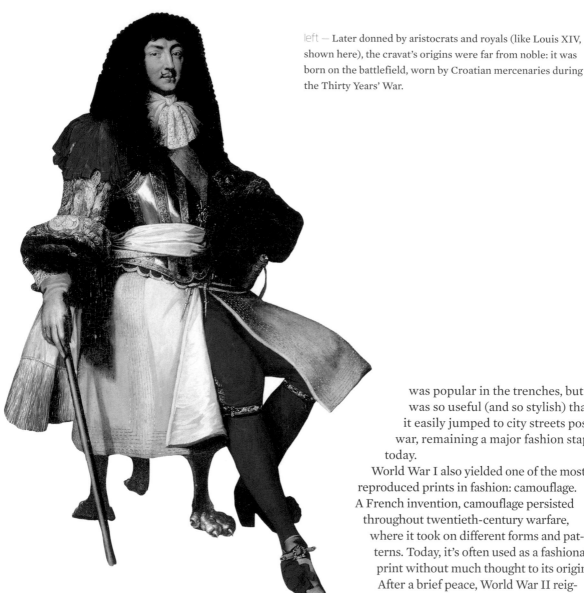

left — Later donned by aristocrats and royals (like Louis XIV, shown here), the cravat's origins were far from noble: it was born on the battlefield, worn by Croatian mercenaries during the Thirty Years' War.

was popular in the trenches, but it was so useful (and so stylish) that it easily jumped to city streets postwar, remaining a major fashion staple today.

World War I also yielded one of the most reproduced prints in fashion: camouflage. A French invention, camouflage persisted throughout twentieth-century warfare, where it took on different forms and patterns. Today, it's often used as a fashionable print without much thought to its origins.

After a brief peace, World War II reignited Europe's tensions, this time with higher stakes and global repercussions: Hitler's Nazis aimed to take over Europe, Japan aimed for empire, and the formerly noninterventionist United States developed atomic weapons. Since this conflict took place at the height of cinema, two of the war's fashion staples, the T-shirt and the bomber jacket, made their way into youth culture via cinematic star turns from American film stars Marlon Brando and James Dean (see "Fashion and Film"). Meanwhile, the fashion press of the time reported on couture's tendency toward designing military-inspired uniforms for women, with broad shoulders

makes claims to its development, but is less associated with the style today.) Prior to the trench coat, Burberry manufactured weather-resistant clothing for people like Roald Amundsen and Ernest Shackleton, early explorers of Antarctica. Burberry's key invention was gabardine, a tightly woven, water-resistant fabric that performed well in harsh climates. World War I offered a particularly grim battle environment—the trenches, which were heavily exposed to the weather, were often muddy, cold, and wet. Burberry's design, a long, belted, waterproof coat,

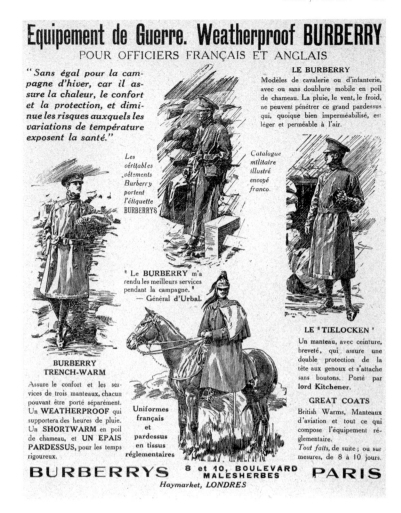

Equipement de Guerre. Weatherproof BURBERRY

POUR OFFICIERS FRANÇAIS ET ANGLAIS

"*Sans égal pour la campagne d'hiver, car il assure la chaleur, le confort et la protection, et diminue les risques auxquels les variations de température exposent la santé.*"

LE BURBERRY

Modèles de cavalerie ou d'infanterie, avec ou sans doublure mobile en poil de chameau. La pluie, le vent, le froid, ne peuvent pénétrer ce grand pardessus qui, quoique bien imperméabilisé, est léger et perméable à l'air.

Les véritables vêtements Burberry portent l'étiquette BURBERRYS

Catalogue militaire illustré envoyé franco.

" *Le* BURBERRY *m'a rendu les meilleurs services pendant la campagne.* " — Général d'Urbal.

BURBERRY TRENCH-WARM

Assure le confort et les services de trois manteaux, chacun pouvant être porté séparément. Un **WEATHERPROOF** qui supportera des heures de pluie. Un **SHORTWARM** en poil de chameau, et **UN EPAIS PARDESSUS**, pour les temps rigoureux.

Uniformes français et pardessus en tissus réglementaires

LE " TIELOCKEN "

Un manteau, avec ceinture, breveté, qui assure une double protection de la tête aux genoux et s'attache sans boutons. Porté par **lord Kitchener**.

GREAT COATS

British Warms, Manteaux d'aviation et tout ce qui compose l'équipement réglementaire. *Tout faits*, de suite ; ou sur mesures, de 8 à 10 jours.

BURBERRYS 8 et 10, BOULEVARD MALESHERBES **PARIS**
Haymarket, LONDRES

and epaulettes. The popularity of these uniform styles was partially an adaptation to wartime rationing: neatly tailored attire took up less fabric than voluminous dresses.

Crucially, for fashion, the German occupation of Paris didn't force the established couture industry, as a whole, to close or relocate (see "Couture"). But the realities of war did change the way things operated. Many couturiers shut down, and some moved: notably, Mainbocher, an American, relocated to New York in 1940, and was commissioned to create the uniforms for the women's division of the Navy, WAVES. A more notorious example is Coco Chanel, who weathered the war as a Nazi sympathizer. She began as German intelligence officer Baron Hans Günther von Dincklage's mistress; the extent of her involvement is uncertain, but some claim that she eventually acted as a Nazi agent. Despite the rumors that swirled around France, Chanel was never punished for her collaboration, and after taking refuge from the controversy in Switzerland for several years, she resumed her couture business in 1953.

Even more notorious were the wartime practices of a German designer whose business still survives today: Hugo Boss. After founding his apparel company in 1924, Boss became a member of the Nazi

above — Sure, a trench coat may suit spring showers, but it was originally meant for much more serious climes: the trenches of World War I.

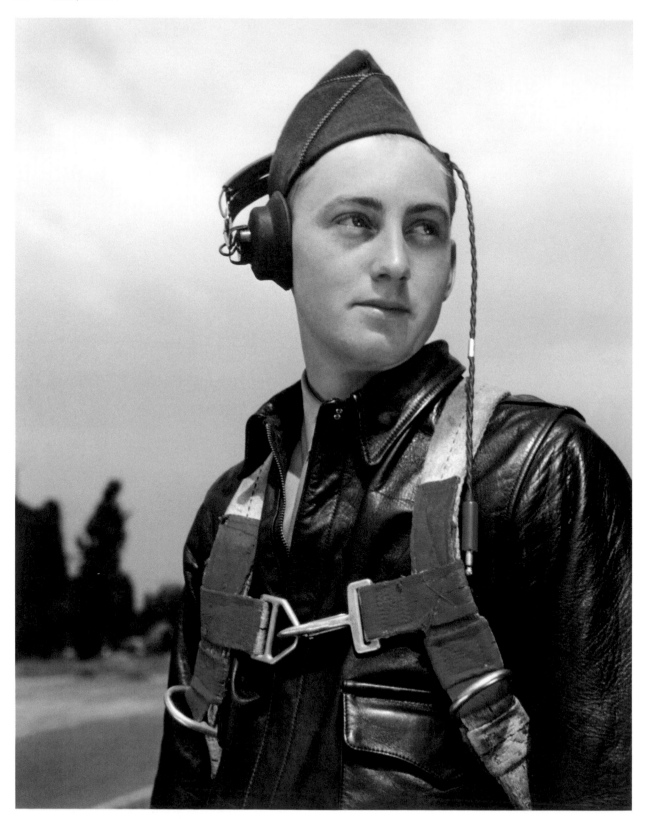

left — GIs were well-acquainted with the bomber jacket before Marlon Brando and James Dean made it a symbol of cool.

right — During World War II, some couturiers contributed to the war effort with design; Mainbocher's uniforms for WAVES, the US Navy's women's division, are a good example.

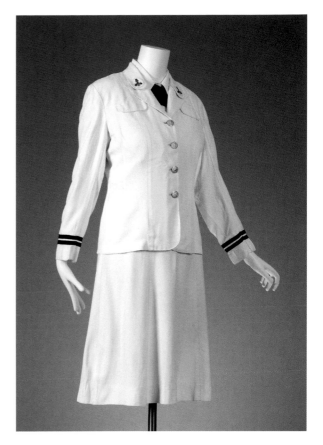

party, and during the war was commissioned to create the German army's uniforms—and did so using forced labor, a fact that didn't come to light until 1997, to much public outrage. Hugo Boss AG, the brand's current incarnation, offered a settlement to survivors in 2001 alongside several other German companies and the German government.

World War II left the world with two great superpowers: the United States and the Soviet Union. Nuclear-armed, politically opposed, and highly paranoid, the two countries became locked in a standoff that became known as the Cold War. One of the Cold War's proxy battles, the Space Race, easily sublimated itself into fashion with the futuristic designs pioneered by André Courrèges in 1964. He was followed by other Space Age designs from Pierre Cardin, Emanuel Ungaro, and Paco Rabanne. Body stockings, pantsuits, minidresses, with liberal use of vinyl and synthetic fabrics, and even the occasional helmet were hallmarks of the look.

With the rise of the rebellious youth culture tied to postwar baby boomers coming of age, the Vietnam War (which began in 1955) quickly became the focus of the pro-peace hippie movement (see "Fashion Subcultures"). With revolutionary figures like Fidel Castro and Ernesto "Che" Guevara as heroes, the hippies appropriated military surplus clothing and wore it to antiwar protests. Tapping into the fervor was Yves Saint Laurent, whose all-black 1968 collection was intended as an antiwar protest. The same year, his safari jacket was featured in a French *Vogue* spread depicting model Veruschka with a gun casually slung across her shoulders, to much controversy. Protest aesthetics also showed up in the designs of Rudi Gernreich for Harmon Knitwear—in the runway show for his 1970 collection, he dressed models in fatigues and army boots and had them carrying guns, a reference to that year's tragedy at Kent State University, where the Ohio National Guard shot students protesting the expansion of the Vietnam War into Cambodia.

Later in the twentieth century, military throwbacks were a recurring theme in fashion. Ralph Lauren's Fall 1990 collection was particularly notable: almost-verbatim copies of World War II uniforms for men and women in olives and tans. The look permeated the nineties, exemplified by the pervasive ads from the Gap featuring choreographed dancers, all in khaki.

Rei Kawakubo's mid-nineties Comme des Garçons collections brought new controversy to military influence. In 1994, Kawakubo chopped up military wear for her collection, drawing criticism for

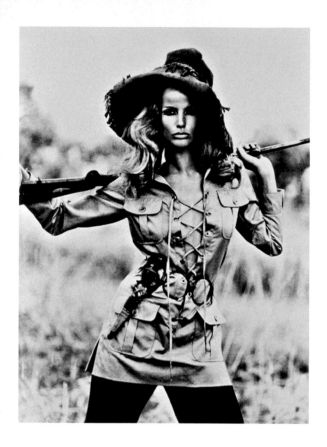

perceived references to the struggle in Bosnia. But this was no match for the scandal she caused in 1995 when she made men's pajamas that resembled Auschwitz prisoner uniforms, a design choice for which she had little explanation. It's one of the more extreme examples of the discomfort that military references in fashion can elicit: using atrocities as fashion inspiration is usually perceived as disrespect.

By the twenty-first century, war took on new meaning with the decentralized violence and paranoia of the War on Terror. Its effects on fashion were seen most dramatically in the immediate wake of 9/11. Up until that point, violent and sadomasochistic images had been a favorite of stylists, photographers, and designers who wanted to shock and create controversy. But with America reeling from a domestic terror attack, fashion magazines and brands rushed to eliminate violent imagery, collections with ominous names, or references to anything dark or threatening. Some, though, chose to take advantage of violent imagery's new ability to shock, most notably Steven Meisel, who shot a story called "State of Emergency" that ran in *Vogue* Italia on the five-year anniversary

of 9/11. A fashion story entirely themed around the War on Terror, the shoot (dubbed "atrocity porn") was heavily controversial; some saw it as glamorizing terrorism, while others viewed it as criticism of the War on Terror.

In the present day, military fashions have staged a major comeback, most visibly with the resurgence of camouflage. The pattern has been everywhere, and in new, creative incarnations on the runway from designers like Patrik Ervell and Dries Van Noten. Van Noten himself claimed he wanted to "demilitarize" camo, which may be difficult, given its pedigree. Even free of criticism or comment, military fashion's influential history is tough to deny.

above — With his antiwar stance, Yves Saint Laurent's custom safari jacket for Veruschka in a 1968 issue of *Vogue* proved to be a loaded statement.

right — By 2013, wildly creative camouflage allowed urbanites to blend in with their stylish surroundings, exemplified by Patrick Ervell's designs.

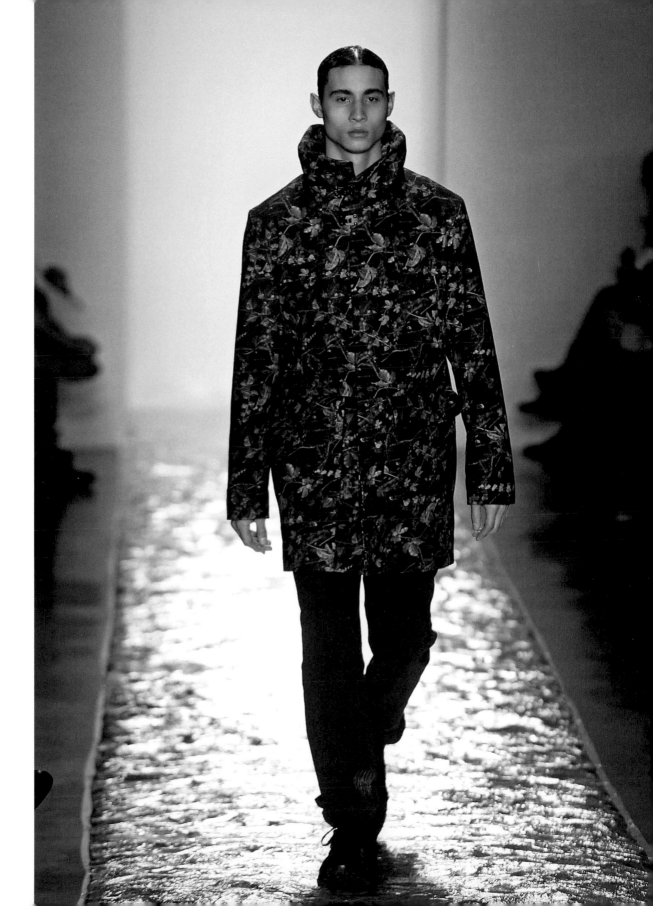

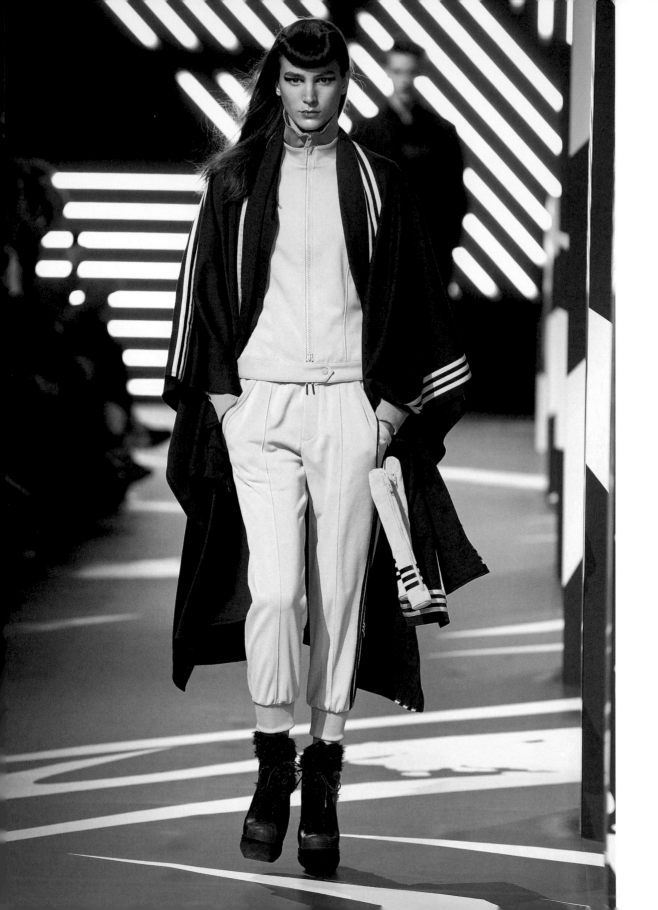

Sports and Fashion

Each summer, tennis greats slip on their all-whites to compete at Wimbledon, the oldest and most prestigious tennis tournament in the world. Media covering the event discuss wins, losses—and even more breathlessly, what the players and spectators wore. In 2013, Serena Williams and Roger Federer donned fashionable white duds from Nike (while Marion Bartoli and Andy Murray won the tournament). Up in the stands, Victoria Beckham wore a slinky Louis Vuitton dress, Jude Law a dapper Ermenegildo Zegna suit. Anna Wintour, fashion's frosty queen, regularly attends; 2013 was no exception, and she was there in Riccardo Tisci. Fashion's relationship with sports, it turns out, is an easy one: in fact, athletic attire was the predecessor of much of today's wardrobe.

Though athleticism has long been a part of human society (look at the Olympic Games), sports as recreation wasn't common until around the time of the Industrial Revolution—coincidentally, the birth of modern fashion (see "Couture"). Much like fashion, leisure sports were originally the domain of the upper classes, and involved the sort of things that one could do on a country estate: riding, hunting, and fishing. These activities required clothing that allowed greater freedom of movement than formal attire did, and it wasn't long before aristocrats cultivated separate city and country wardrobes. One of the first trends sparked by these leisure activities was the "redingote," the French translation of the English riding coat that first became popular in the late eighteenth century. Close fitting and neatly tailored, it was worn by both women and men. Another example is the Norfolk jacket, a single-breasted tweed coat made for shooting and other active pursuits, named after the Duke of Norfolk and popularized by Edward VII. It was a staple in middle-class wardrobes by the 1880s.

The popularity of aristocratic leisurewear also provided a boost to the tailoring business. The most dramatic example lies in the history of the British couture label House of Redfern. Originally a draper, John Redfern opened his first shop in Cowes, on the Isle of Wight. Serendipitously, Cowes transformed into a hotspot for that most upper crust of leisure sports, yachting, and by 1871 Redfern smartly expanded his offerings to tailored yachting attire

left — Yohji Yamamoto's form is impeccable in his collaboration with Adidas, Y-3, which brings an avant-garde edge to athletic wear. Shown here: Y-3's Fall/Winter 2014–15 collection.

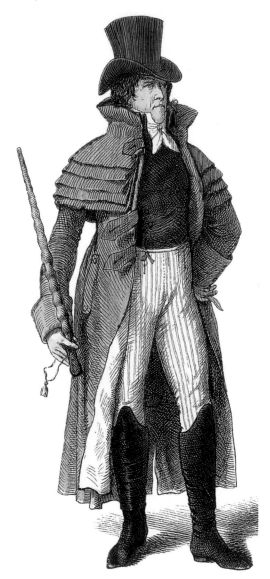

for women. His sporting clothes proved extremely popular, and were featured in *Harper's Bazaar*; these successes led Redfern to design couture.

Tailored sportswear may have come courtesy of the aristocracy, but equally as influential were schools and their legacy of team sports. Sports that resembled football were played in English private schools as early as the fifteenth century, but it wasn't until the early nineteenth century that these sports were truly codified—and with the rules came the uniforms. One lasting contribution to modern wardrobes is the rugby jersey, first worn at the English school Rugby in 1939. The striped shirt with a collar is still recognizable as a rugby uniform today, both

on fields and in fashion—notably, Ralph Lauren designs rugby-inspired attire for everyday wear. But the rugby jersey is far from team sports' only contribution to fashion. Another key piece is the sweater, a knit wool overlayer used to keep players warm, which worked its way into couture in Chanel's 1920s designs (see "Couture").

At the same time as team sports were flourishing in England, America's signature sport was taking shape: baseball. The game first appeared in New York in 1846, but the first uniforms were worn by the Cincinnati Red Stockings, who in 1868 paired loose knee breeches, known as knickerbockers, with knee socks, a shirt, and a cap with a brim—very much the baseball uniform of today. Baseball uniforms influenced activewear for other sports, while

above — Like its name suggests, the redingote (riding coat) was made for horseback riding and other leisure activities, bringing menswear greater informality.

right — When yachting brought the gentry to Cowes, local tailor John Redfern took advantage of the situation, landing his designs in the pages of magazines like *La Gazette du Bon Ton* (shown here, from 1913) and *Harper's Bazaar*.

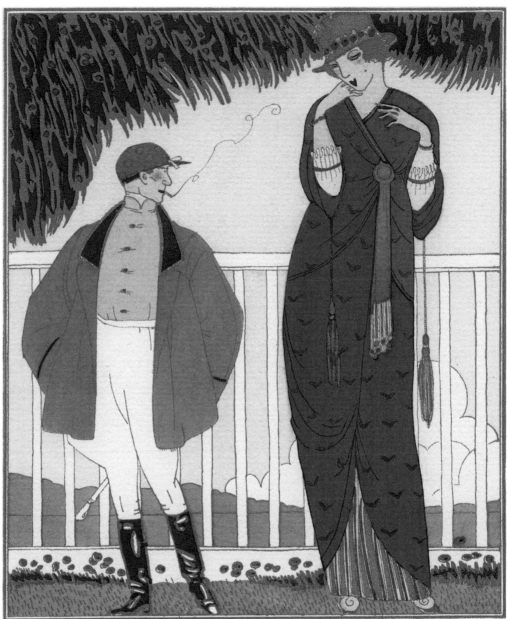

VOUS DITES... CANCAN II

Robe pour les courses de Redfern

the baseball cap became a fashion classic, reaching its peak popularity later in the twentieth century. By the 1920s, everyday clothing styles became a little less formal, and this spirit transformed the tennis court. French tennis star René Lacoste introduced the pique tennis shirt to the court at the 1926 US Open, creating a stir with his innovative on-court attire. He founded his own clothing company in 1933, famously creating the trademark alligator logo shirt that became so popular with the American "preppies" of the seventies and eighties. Around the same time as Lacoste was active, the first female tennis star, Suzanne Lenglen, was scandalizing audiences with her bare forearms and short skirts designed by the couturier Patou. Following in the footsteps of Lacoste, meanwhile, was Fred Perry, an English Wimbledon champ. Perry began manufacturing tennis shirts similar to Lacoste's in the forties, with a wreath logo. Notably, Fred Perry shirts became popular with the mods of the fifties (see "Subcultures"), whose obsession with the shirts prompted the brand to produce it in colors beyond the classic white.

Sportswear had become America's special domain within fashion design by the thirties, with designers like Claire McCardell pioneering the field. The term is somewhat misleading: sportswear came to mean casual, ready-to-wear ensembles, not clothing intended for sports. So-called sportswear takes its name from that traditional divide between city clothes and country clothes from the nineteenth century: back then, the only casual clothing was for genteel sports like hunting and riding. These days, the term "sportswear" continues to denote what is simply casual attire—but the influence of sports on fashion continues, unabated.

After World War II, the rise of youth culture (see "Fashion Subcultures") prompted a huge shift in the way people dressed: formality was out, informality was in. With their active lifestyles, youths were drawn to athletic attire, integrating it into their wardrobes: suddenly, sports shoes were fashionable. Around the same time, the rise of movies and television accelerated the development of celebrity culture (see "Celebrity Fashion"), which easily embraced sports stars as style idols. The most popular sports celebrities were usually those with a unique style of play that compelled audiences. One

right — The first female tennis celebrity, Suzanne Lenglen dazzled and shocked audiences with her on-court domination, off-court antics, and revealing Patou tennis dresses.

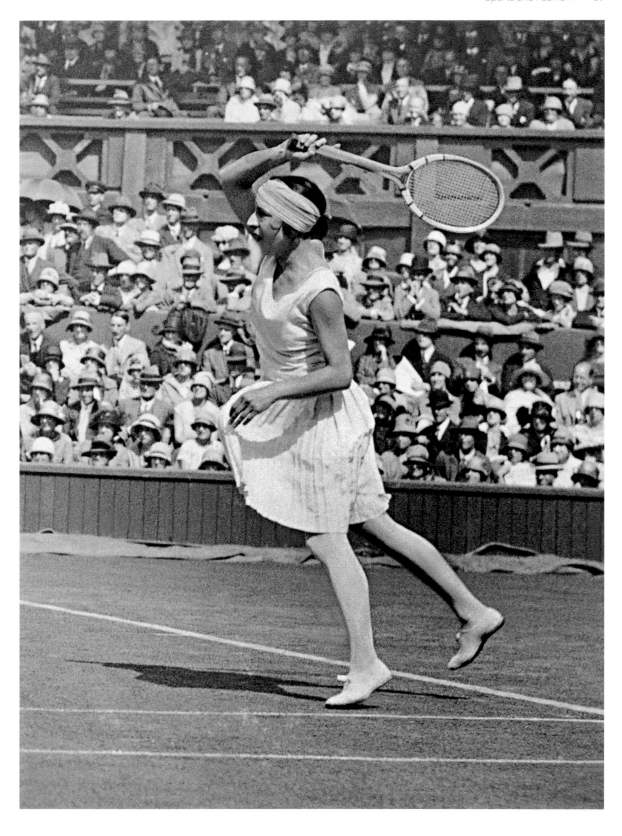

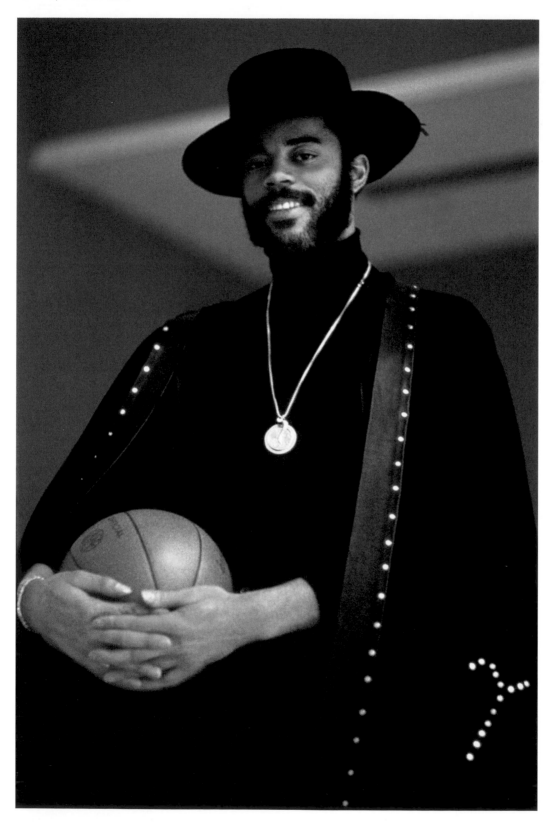

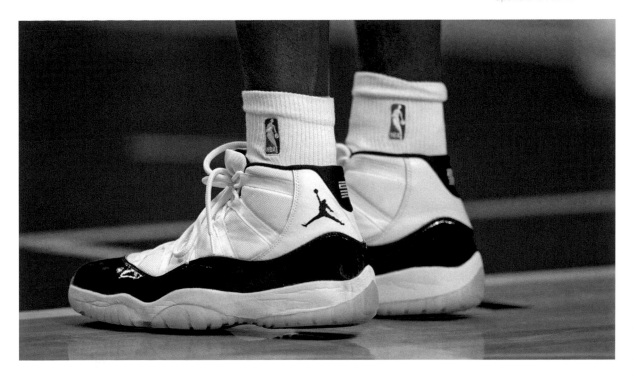

of the earliest examples is George Best, a Manchester United footballer whose Swinging-Sixties fashion-forward style and charisma on and off the field inspired public adulation. Conscious of his sartorial influence, he became the proprietor of clothing boutiques in Manchester. His role as a style icon foreshadows the later (and much wider) influence of one of the biggest sports icons of the early twenty-first century, David Beckham.

By the seventies, a more flamboyant fashionability appeared in another sport: basketball. New York Knicks star Walt "Clyde" Frazier received his nickname for sporting a hat like Warren Beatty's in *Bonnie and Clyde*, and was widely known for his outré fashion sense, favoring flashy suits, mink coats,

left — Full of bravado both on the court and off, Walt "Clyde" Frazier's flamboyant style (shown here in 1973) earned him the first sports celebrity shoe.

above — By the 1980s and 1990s, Air Jordans (shown on-court here in 1995) were such a hot commodity that wearers risked being mugged for their footwear.

and ostentatious feathered hats. By 1974, Puma had manufactured the very first celebrity basketball shoe for Frazier—the Puma Clyde, a suede shoe with a gold signature on the side. The shoe was quickly embraced by the burgeoning hip-hop subculture, which claimed athletic wear as its sartorial marker (see "Fashion and Music" for how Run-DMC popularized Adidas). But the Clyde wasn't the last celebrity basketball shoe: in the eighties, Air Jordans, named for superstar Chicago Bulls player Michael Jordan, were introduced by Nike. This was the beginning of the era of fashionable trainers, with every teenager clamoring to own a pair—the shoes were so sought-after that some people mugged and even murdered wearers who wouldn't give up their precious shoes. Around the same time, another sports basic had been channeled into mainstream fashion via the conduit of hip-hop: baseball caps. By the late eighties, newspapers enthusiastically reported how the caps were trendy (brim backwards was the edgiest), with high-fashion versions produced by labels like Chanel.

By the late twentieth century, some newly popular sports were developing their own subcultures. One was skateboarding, which emerged in the seventies, but had its most notable impacts on fashion when it moved from skateparks to the streets in the nineties. That decade saw an explosion of skate shoe brands like Etnies, Airwalk, and Vans, as well as the debut of Supreme, which moved from producing skate clothes in 1994 to attain more mainstream popularity in the early aughts. Much of this mainstreaming of skate fashion can be credited to the popularity of pro skaters like Mark Gonzales and Tony Hawk. Around the same time, yoga was rising as a sport of choice for young, mostly female urbanites seeking a heady mix of spirituality and flexibility. By the twenty-first century, yoga studios were seemingly popping up by the dozens in every city, while yogawear made its way onto the street. One brand to emerge as a style leader was founded in 1998. Lululemon transformed the original stretchy yoga pant into something trendier and more fashionable, and soon Lululemon pants were cluttering closets everywhere, often as a substitute for "real" pants.

A final sign of the fashion world's thrall to athleticism is the ascendance of designer collaborations with athletic wear brands. One of the most notable is Y-3, avant-garde Japanese designer Yohji Yamamoto's partnership with Adidas (see "Global Fashion"), which debuted in 2003. Y-3 has given Adidas the sort of high-fashion clout it wouldn't normally have, while lending Yamamoto room to experiment. Also successful has been Stella McCartney's line of women's sportswear for Adidas—not as provocative as Y-3, but still popular. Meanwhile, Puma started Puma Black Label to bring a more design-forward aesthetic to the company, even tapping Alexander McQueen for a collaboration. If there were any doubts of Puma's seriousness about fashion, the brand's hiring of edgy designer Hussein Chalayan as creative director in 2008 dispelled them.

And this is the world we live in today: the sportswear of past years is mainstream fashion, current athletic wear is fashion inspiration, and high-end fashion designers get press for creating fancy running shoes. It's little wonder the fashion photographers at Wimbledon don't stop at the stands: the court is where fashion begins.

right — These days, fashionable yogawear isn't a stretch. From yoga studios to city streets, Lululemons are ubiquitous.

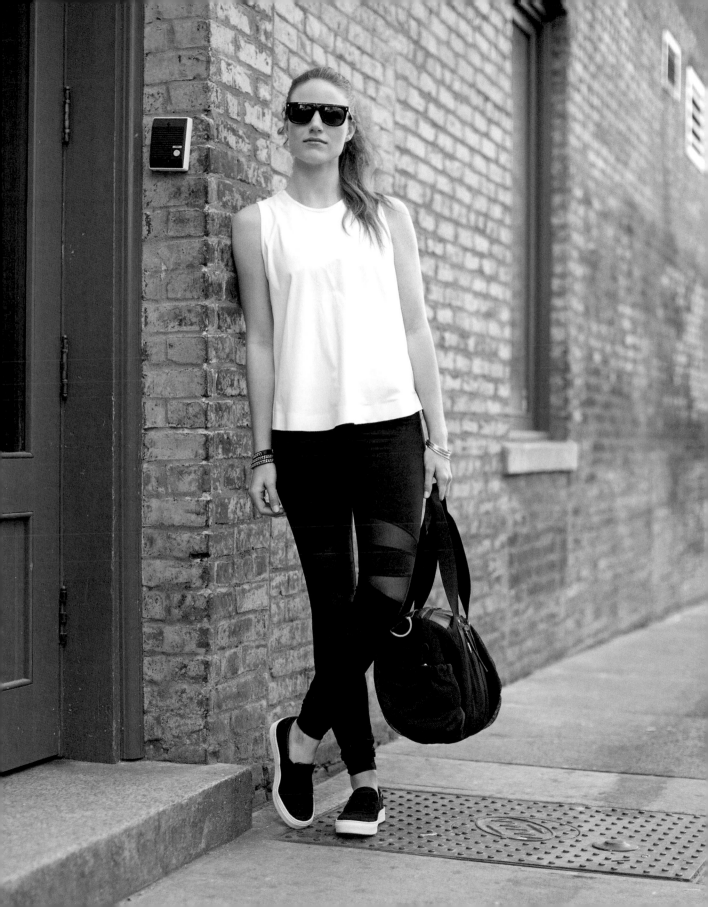

Menswear

Drinking whiskey, seducing women, and doing it all in a well-tailored suit: on TV's *Mad Men*, Don Draper is the archetype of masculinity, and his suit is a big part of that. A sharp suit holds a special symbolic power in Western culture's aesthetic language: a man wearing one is absolutely a *man*. But men's style didn't begin with the suit, and one only needs to glance at newsstands today, replete with menswear titles like *Complex*, *GQ*, and *Details*, to know that it won't end there, either. Menswear hasn't always been a somber affair. If you rewind time to the era of Louis XIV (see "Royal Fashion"), the fashion-obsessed Sun King who reigned during the seventeenth and early eighteenth centuries, men's attire was openly peacocky. Trousers weren't yet in style. A typical outfit included loose breeches called "petticoat breeches," so named because they resembled women's petticoats, paired with stockings. The look was finished with a flourish of decorative ribbons tied around the waist. Long hair and curled wigs were de rigueur. Louis XIV himself was a showboat, and his decadent attire, made to befit his role of absolute power, included high heels to accentuate his legs. Soon after the French Revolution, men's fashion made a dramatic shift toward the practical, the restrained, the muted—a transition dubbed "the

Great Male Renunciation" by psychoanalyst John Flügel. This paring down is sometimes attributed to the anti-aristocratic revolutionary fervor of the French Revolution, but it really had more to do with the Industrial Revolution, which was first felt keenly in London. The Industrial Revolution led to the rise of the middle class and workers' social mobility, and so the attire of the working man, the suit, became fashionable. At the same time, the British aristocracy's increasing involvement with country life and its sporting activities (see "Sports and Fashion"), and their habit of spending the "social season" in the city, brought clothing made for activities such as riding and hunting into greater popularity—and fueled the early success of the tailors of Savile Row. By the end of the eighteenth century, the English and the French had two distinct styles of menswear. The English look was more tailored, involving riding coats, breeches, and riding caps and boots, while the French look was slimmer-fitting

right — James Bond never goes out of style; neither does his tuxedo. Here, Pierce Brosnan appears as the secret service agent in 1997.

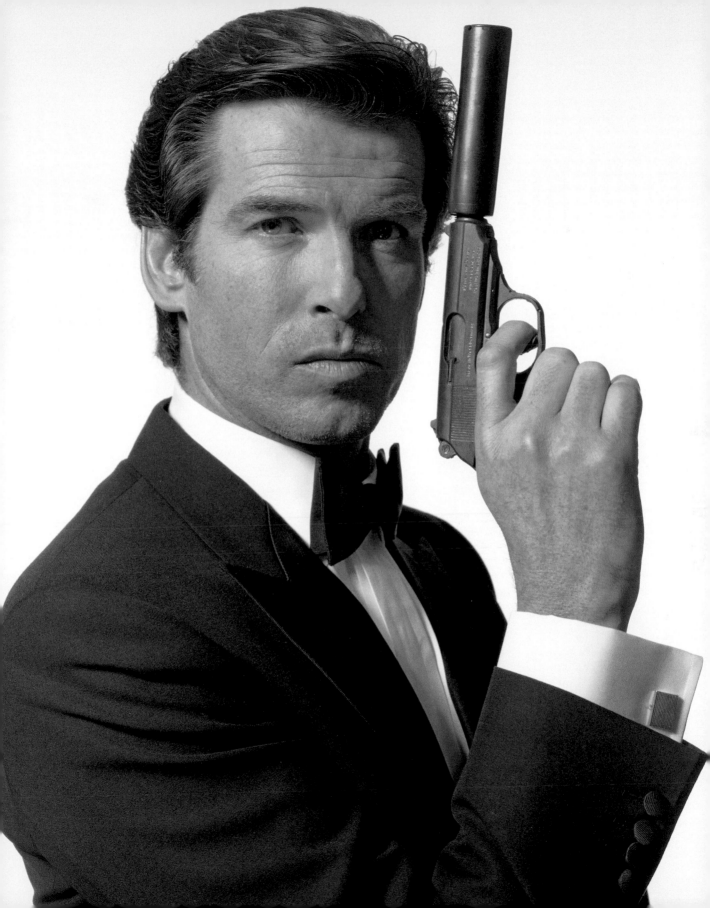

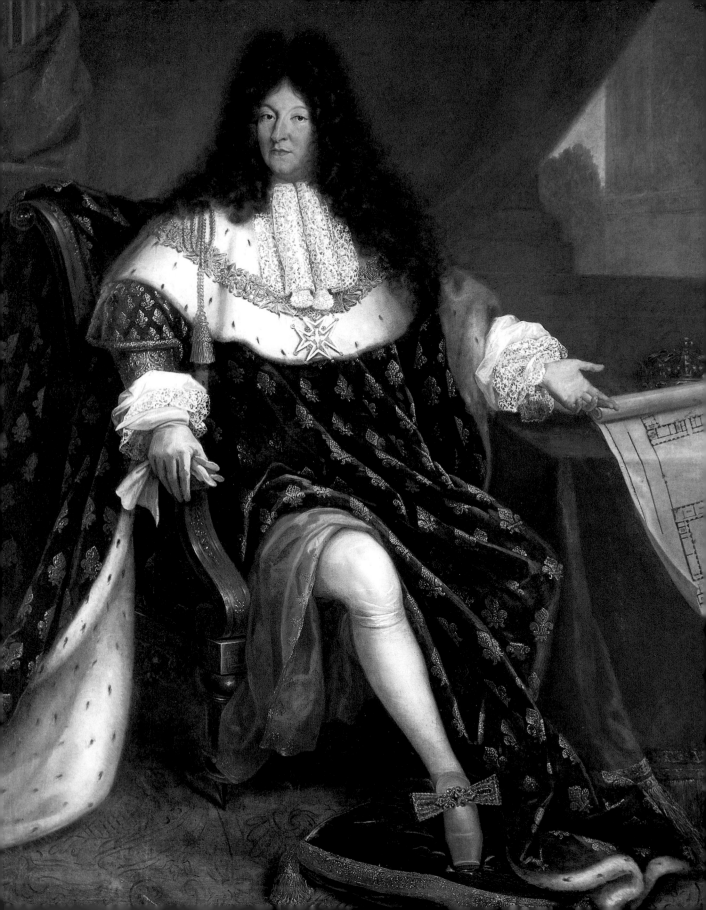

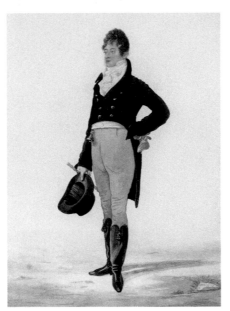 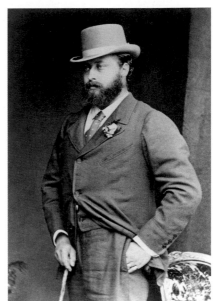

and more ostentatious, consisting of tight waistcoats paired with short skirts and breeches.

The first group of men to truly exploit this sartorial dichotomy were the macaronis of late eighteenth-century England. A subclass of fops, fashionable men often ridiculed for their sartorial interest, the classic macaroni was a well-traveled young man who brought continental styles home with him. But the style expanded, and soon macaroni fashions were available in all price ranges. Macaronis wore rich fabrics and pastels with metallic flourishes, paired with red-heeled shoes, tall wigs, and swords.

left —In the seventeenth century, men dressed to impress: here, French King Louis XIV shows he's no wallflower with opulent robes, luxurious tights, and flowing tresses.

above left — Stylish men today can thank the very first dandy, Beau Brummell (pictured in 1805), for bringing a trim, tailored aesthetic to menswear in the late eighteenth and early nineteenth centuries.

above right — Queen Victoria's son Edward VII (shown here in 1870) wore a black dinner jacket that ushered in that icon of formal menswear, the tuxedo.

The ostentatious dress inspired mockery; the most famous example is the song "Yankee Doodle Dandy," which used the term "macaroni" to insinuate that the colonials were effeminate.

While macaronis clearly sprang from the French style of dressing, another group took the English style to a new level of fashionability: the dandies. The very first dandy was Beau Brummell, easily the most influential man of style in the late eighteenth and early nineteenth century. Brummell used clothing for a clear purpose: to endear himself to the upper classes and society at large through dress and presentation, an uncommon feat at a time when class determined almost everything.

Brummell's social climbing began in the military. Britain's standing army was built during the mid-seventeenth century, and with it came standardized military uniforms. So enamored was Brummell with military sartorial conventions that he used military tailors to make his civilian clothes, which included a notable item: pantaloons, the first long trousers for men. His typical outfit included slender pantaloons, starched shirts with a high collar, a coat, and a cravat—the precursor to the modern necktie. His look was tailored and understated, a polished version of the English style of dress. Brummell paraded around town, attended all the right parties, and positioned

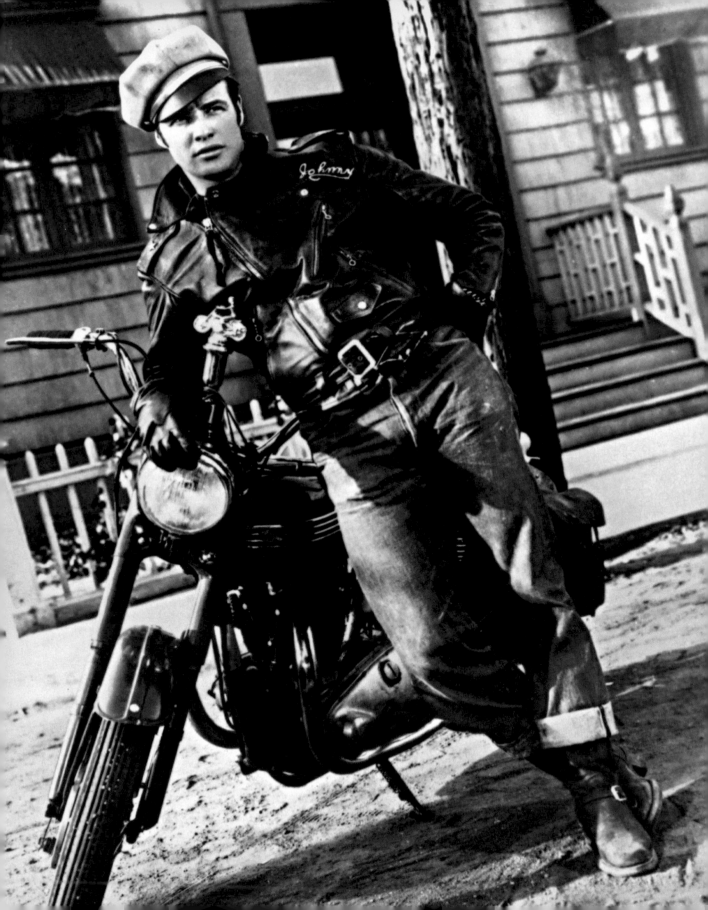

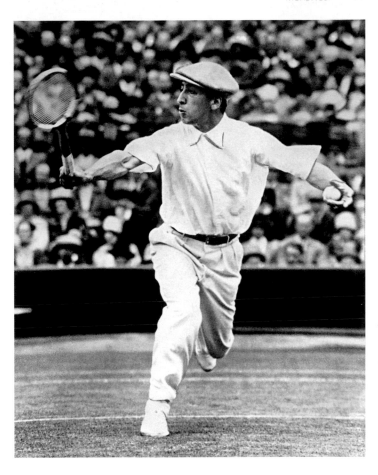

himself to be seen. His look caught on, spurring business for the tailors of Savile Row. The ensuing trend inspired much speculation and analysis, including by Charles Baudelaire, who considered dandyism's relentless pursuit of aesthetics as almost a kind of spirituality—while others regarded dandies as bored, vapid slaves to style. Regardless, the clean lines and crisp tailoring of Brummell's dandyism have influ-

left — Marlon Brando's bad-boy style in *The Wild One* inspired copycats, and soon black leather jackets and blue jeans were symbols of everyday sartorial rebellion.

above — French tennis star René Lacoste (photographed at Wimbledon in 1928) made an impression with his on-court style, and the pique tennis shirt became a menswear smash.

enced the form of stylish men's clothing ever since. Since Brummell's time, the suit has refined itself by slowly stripping away complexity, a combined result of society's increasing informality as well as men's growing need for mobility to pursue sports like hunting, fishing, and riding. The long Victorian frock coat yielded to the less formal morning jacket, eventually giving way, during the Edwardian era, to the even less formal lounge suit, today known as a business suit. The Prince of Wales (before he became Edward VII) was somewhat responsible for the creation of the tuxedo, after he requested a black dinner jacket modeled after a smoking jacket. He introduced the idea to an American businessman in 1886, who took the look back to his affluent New York State village of Tuxedo Park. A modified version of this suit took the village's name, and it stuck. Ever since, the tux has been the definition of formal men's attire, eventually enshrined in culture by its representation in James Bond films in the twentieth and twenty-first centuries.

Twentieth-century menswear has been variously shaped by sports, wars, and popular culture. Early in the century, sportswear moved beyond the precise tailoring of hunting and fishing clothes to influence casual wear (see "Sports and Fashion"). One pivotal moment came at the US Open in 1926, when French tennis star René Lacoste debuted a practical style that allowed him more movement on the court: the pique tennis shirt. The tennis shirt was also introduced to polo and golf, and became one of the staples of casual menswear. Professional sports continues to influence men's fashion in many ways: baseball jackets, sneakers, and of course the ubiquitous baseball cap all come from professional sports. The twentieth century's two history-changing wars also had a huge impact on menswear, including new styles brought about by the military's innovations in battle attire (see "Wars and Military Fashion"). One example is the trench coat, a garment made to withstand the harsh conditions of the trenches during World War I. The long, belted, waterproof coat is claimed as an invention of both Aquascutum and Burberry, but the latter is certainly more identified with this iconic jacket today.

World War II, meanwhile, brought two particularly notable inventions to male attire: black leather jackets and white T-shirts. While they were all too familiar to GIs, it was really the movies that brought tees and leather jackets mainstream appeal in the wardrobes of Marlon Brando and James Dean for *The Wild One* (1953) and *Rebel Without a Cause* (1955), respectively. In these roles, the two bad-boy screen icons made another pivotal style decision: to wear blue jeans. Though jeans had long been considered workwear, Brando and Dean made these tough cotton trousers a staple of a rebellious young man's wardrobe. By the seventies, jeans became less edgy—they were everywhere, worn by everybody.

Like womenswear, menswear was forever changed by the informal fashions and the pursuit of individuality that accompanied youth culture's triumph in the sixties (see "Fashion Subcultures" and "Fashion and Music"). Music was hugely influential: the Beatles, with their distinctive haircuts and mod-influenced suits, inspired imitation. By the seventies,

right — In the 1970s, menswear copied some moves from the dance floor, and tighter, flashier clothes like those worn by John Travolta in 1977's *Saturday Night Fever* hit the streets.

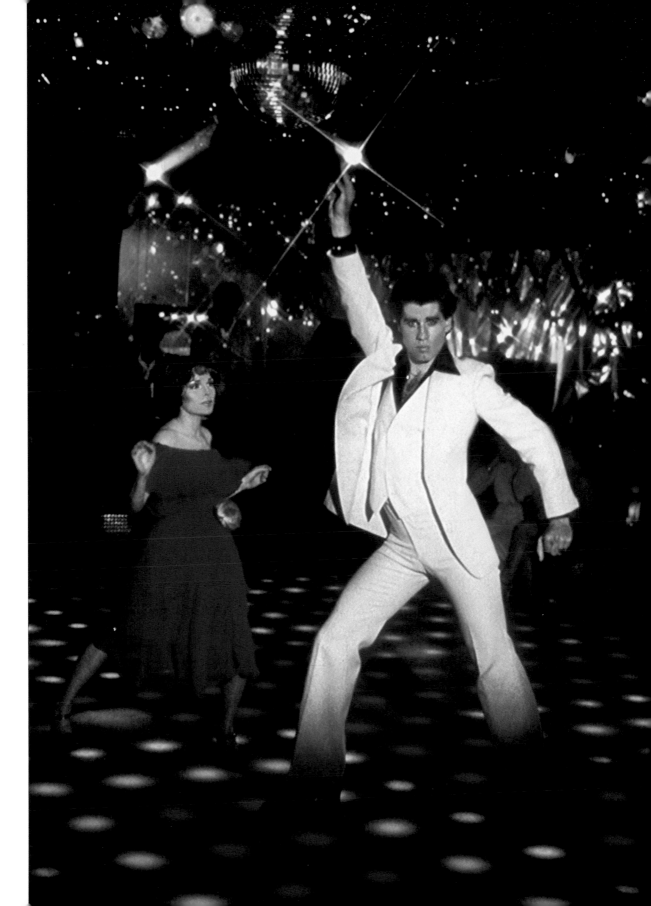

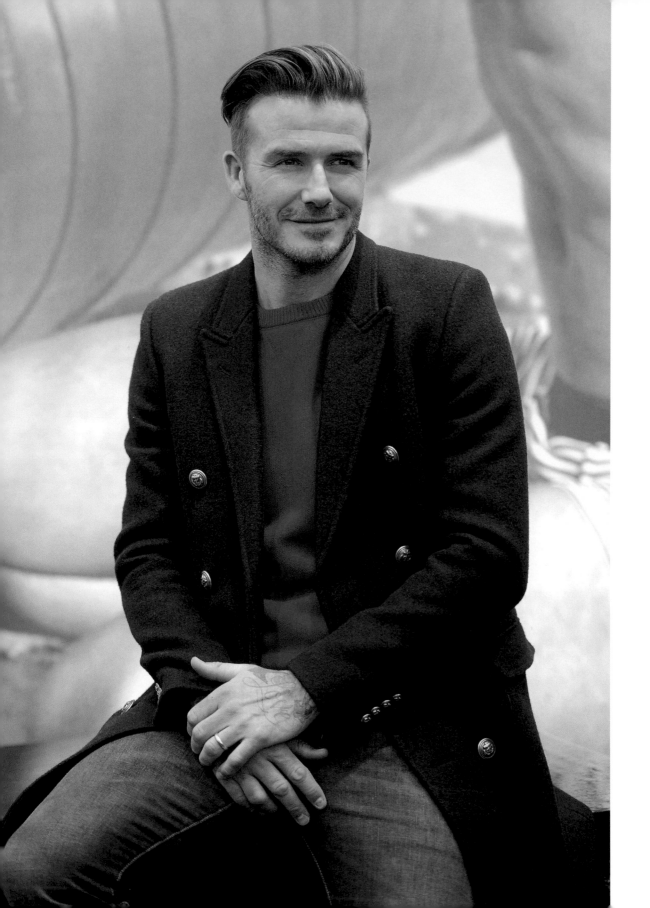

the three-piece suits and bellbottoms of the disco scene infected men's closets with a little *Saturday Night Fever*. But when it comes to modern menswear, the biggest influence has come from hip-hop and rap, with their penchant for sportswear. The look began in the early eighties with Run-DMC, who took Adidas tracksuits and sneakers and made them cool. Today's casual menswear is very much indebted to hip-hop's early style choices, while modern rap and hip-hop stars like Kanye West and Pharrell Williams are top arbiters of style.

Another development of the eighties was the rise of the "new man," for whom fashion-consciousness was an acceptable thing. The new man was born from the women's movement (see "Feminism and Fashion") that aimed to bring equality to the workforce, and in so doing forced men to redefine their masculinity. As this happened, men's fashion became a major concern. The appetite for fashionable male apparel and grooming products expanded, male models took over the fashion runways, and men's fashion magazines began to proliferate, including a redesigned *GQ*, which has been credited with giving the newly fashion-conscious,

body-conscious male media representation. By the nineties, this man had a new name: the metrosexual. TV shows like *Queer Eye for the Straight Guy* capitalized on the trend, molding men into metrosexuals with the help of fashion-conscious gay men (see "Gay and Lesbian Fashion"). Well-groomed, well-sculpted men rose to the top of the entertainment industry, including one who became the icon of metrosexual masculinity: David Beckham. An impeccably styled soccer player, Beckham's overwhelming physical beauty and fashion consciousness have brought him celebrity status and modeling gigs, including a recurring role as an underwear model for brands like Calvin Klein and H&M. He has seen his contemporary successor in the sensitive and well-styled Ryan Gosling.

In the twenty-first century, we've seen the rise of the modern dandy: the hipster. As apolitical and image conscious as their dandy predecessors, hipsters have been responsible for reintroducing some retro menswear traditions to the mainstream: slim-cut trousers and jeans, barbered hair, thick-framed glasses, and artisanal everything.

Today, the men's clothing industry is booming—and despite the Great Male Renunciation and the sober lines of the suit, men's fashionable attire is varied. Walking through any major city, you'll see men dressed in everything from hip hop-inspired sportswear, to edgy leather jackets, to designer jeans—and sometimes, yes, a plain black suit.

left — He began as a footballer, but David Beckham's surefooted style made him a fashion icon; in this photo, he promotes his underwear line for H&M in early 2014.

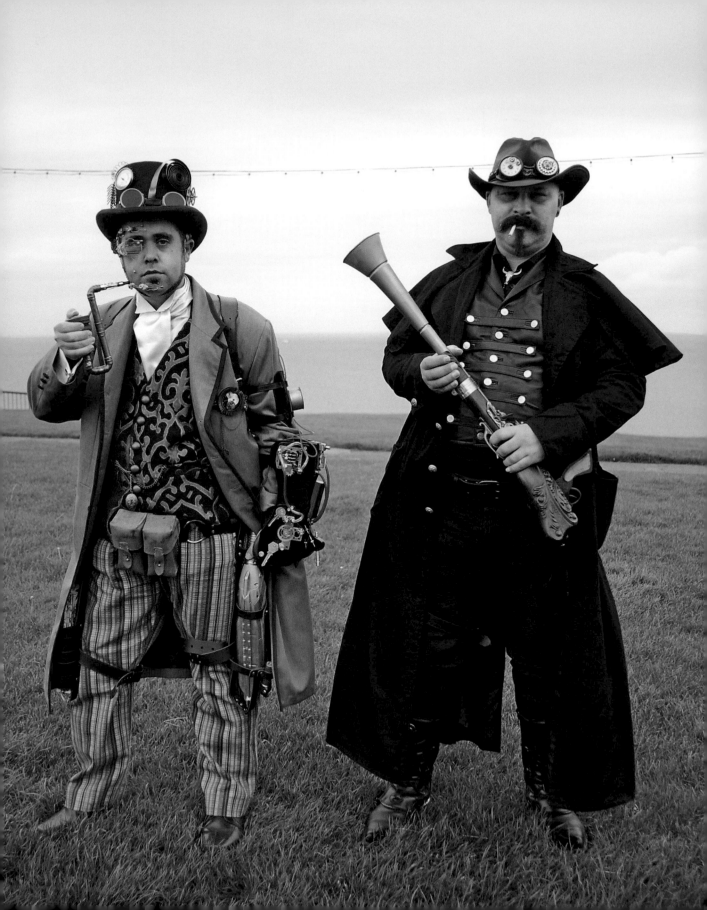

Fashion Subcultures

Punk was the unlikely theme of 2013's Met Ball, inspired by the exhibition *Punk: Chaos to Couture* at the Metropolitan Museum of Art's Costume Institute. In between all the red carpet posing, the gala inspired a lot of mockery: many of the guests (celebrities, socialites, and fashion types) wore couture duds that didn't live up to the theme, and Vivienne Westwood, the queen of punk fashion, was barely addressed by the press. But the whole shindig may have been doomed to failure from the start: punk subculture is dedicated to undermining the mainstream and overthrowing the corporate—and what's more mainstream, more corporate, than the Met Ball?

Subcultures have been the barnacles on mainstream fashion's belly throughout the twentieth century. Springing up as a reaction to mainstream culture, subcultures use fashion as a way to create a distinct identity. Often (but not always) associated with music (see "Fashion and Music"), subcultures are usually youth-driven; in fact, they're a largely post-Industrial Revolution invention, coinciding with children being kept longer in school and thus staying under their parents' care after puberty. Naturally, these proto-adults sought a way to rebel, and subcultures were the result.

One of the first subcultures to truly take hold of fashion was that of the flapper. Flappers were emancipated women who emerged after getting a taste of the work force during World War I. Flappers drank, danced the Charleston in jazz clubs, and boasted a very distinct style: short, bobbed haircuts, drop-waist dresses, flat chests, and short skirts. Called the "garçonne look," in high fashion it became associated with Coco Chanel. But when the Great Depression hit in 1929, the indulgent flapper lifestyle became a thing of the past.

In the wake of flappers, a male fashion subculture rose to the fore: zoot suiters (see "Menswear"). Zoot suiters weren't a homologous group, but the uniform—a dramatically cut suit featuring wide shoulders and billowing trousers that tapered at the knee—became worn by African Americans as well as a particular Latin American subculture, the pachuco. Pachucos emerged in El Paso, Texas in the thirties, and were known for their well-dressed, flamboyant style. They became infamous after the Zoot Suit

left — Steampunk is definitely not dead: the subculture, which fuses old timey details with sci-fi futurism, inspires cultish devotion. Shown here are two steampunks at the Whitby Gothic Weekend in 2013.

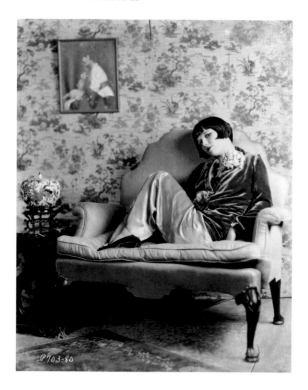

Riots of 1943 in Los Angeles, when military service-men clashed with the pachucos, offended by the way they scandalously flouted wartime rationing with their fabric-heavy attire.

Teddy Boys, meanwhile, were a bit of a throwback. Labeled by the *New York Times* as "Britain's Zoot Suiters" in 1954, Teddy Boys were the first subculture rooted in nostalgia. Formally called "Edwardians" and nicknamed "Teddy Boys" by a distrustful media, Teddies were young, working-class men who dressed up in styles once worn by their Edwardian dandy grandfathers: fancy vests, drainpipe trousers, velvet collars, and long hair swept up into a pompadour. Labeled as delinquents, the Teddy Boys had a strong influence on men's subcultural fashion in Britain going forward, particularly the mods of the fifties and sixties, who were known for their fastidious fashionability, made-to-measure suits, and scooters. Contrasting with the dapper, consumer-focused mods were the rockers, who wore leather jackets and jeans, and rode motorcycles. The two subcultures, with their opposing looks and outlooks, couldn't stand each other, and regularly brawled, inspiring public hysteria in Britain.

Across the ocean, in the United States of the forties, another influential subculture was taking shape: the Beat Generation. The Beats (supposedly coined by Jack Kerouac) first appeared in Greenwich Village, and flaunted a bohemian lifestyle steeped in edgy literature, poetry readings, marijuana, and jazz. The Beats cultivated a look, too: long hair, turtlenecks, sandals, and a lot of the color black. The media became obsessed with the Beats, however, and turned their look into a cliché that was rolled out at costume parties; in 1958 a newspaper reporter renamed them "beatniks," a pejorative nickname that Allen Ginsberg publically detested. But the name stuck, and the look, stereotype or not, worked its way into fashion, including the collections of Yves Saint Laurent.

The Beats were the spiritual predecessors of the hippies. Hippies are arguably youth culture's most

above — With her bobbed hair and wanton ways, film star Louise Brooks (pictured here in 1928) exemplified the flapper lifestyle.

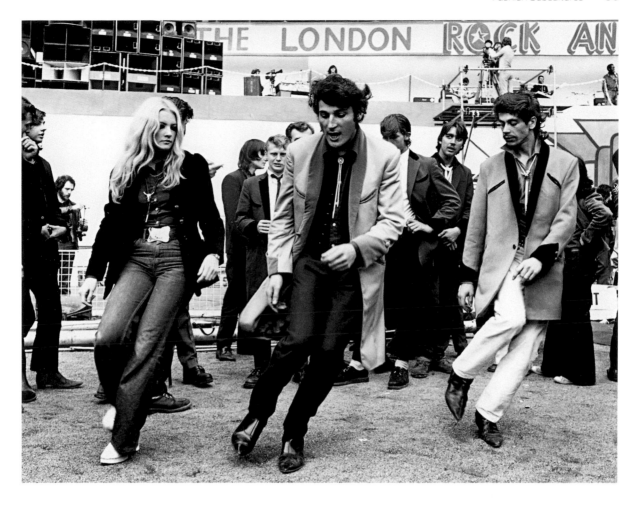

celebrated subculture, the result of large numbers of Baby Boomers who all came of age at once. The hippies had causes: they opposed the Vietnam War, championed racial equality, and embraced sexual freedom. They believed in natural lifestyles, Mother Earth, Eastern philosophy—and took psychedelic drugs to expand their minds. Their fashion reflected all this: a nonconformist assortment of thrift-store finds and non-Western clothing (dashikis, saris, and the like), bell-bottoms, sandals, beads, leather vests,

above — Though the sharp-dressed Teddy Boys (shown here dancing at Wembley Arena) borrowed their style from the buttoned-up Edwardian era, they had a reputation for being wild.

and trippy patterns like tie-dye. The hippies continued with their sit-ins and love-ins until the end of the sixties, when the double blow of Altamont's Hells Angels-driven violence and the Manson Family murders brought the era of peace and love to a shocking end. Hippie fashions, however, live on into the present, inspiring looks from music festivals to high-fashion runways.

Youth culture's collective loss of innocence spawned a subculture with a particularly hard edge: punk (see "Music and Fashion"). Punk appeared in New York and London in the seventies, and the look and lifestyle were wound up inextricably with punk music and bands like the Sex Pistols and the Ramones. Spiked hair, piercings, studded belts, and torn shirts were a symbolic middle finger to society, an embodiment of the subculture's antiestablishment attitude.

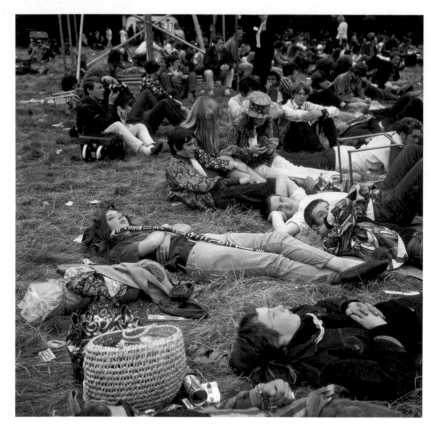

left — Peace, love, and tie-dye: the hippie style embraced a nonconformist, psychedelic, bohemian aesthetic, as shown in this photo of a 1967 love-in.

The look spawned legions of imitators (often derided as "poseurs"), and punk's legitimacy has been an issue ever since, exemplified by the song "Punk Is Dead" by Crass: "Ain't for revolution, it's just for cash / Punk became a fashion just like hippy used to be / Ain't got a thing to do with you or me."

In the wake of punk's theoretical selling out, goth delivered the kind of depressed, apolitical subculture the disenfranchised youth needed. Springing from the music scene led by bands like Bauhaus, the goth look was all-black, romantic, sometimes involving Victorian or Edwardian garb, and often religious or occult symbols. As a subculture without a real cause, besides being a refuge for depressed youth, goth hasn't suffered quite the same identity crisis as punk, and when its looks appear in collections by people such as Alexander McQueen or Jean Paul Gaultier, it's just another ebony feather in goth's black hat.

The eighties saw the popularization of hip-hop subculture, which blossomed in the Bronx in the seventies with the creative, underground competition of graffiti, rap, and breakdancing. Tracksuits and sneakers by brands like Adidas and Converse became popular. Like punk and goth, hip-hop style was popularized via music, with the coming of the music video and MTV being particularly important in spreading the look.

By the nineties, dance music was on a high, reaching its apex in rave culture. Rave really began in the eighties, in the clubs of Manchester, but it spread around the globe, attaining mass popularity by the mid-nineties. Since their all-night drug-fueled dance parties were illegal and usually held in secluded spaces such as abandoned warehouses or fields in the middle of nowhere, ravers attained an almost tribal sense of unity expressed by their mantra, PLUR: peace, love, unity, respect. Ravers wore a particular variety of club clothes: phat pants, which were swimmingly wide, bigger at the ankle than the waist, and shirts made from shiny fabrics; or, often

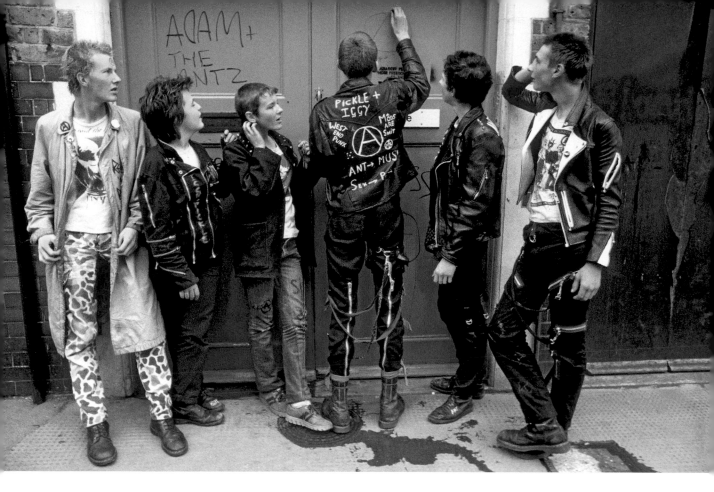

for girls, baby tees and pigtails and rainbow-colored accessories (a style called "candy raver"). Common accessories included pacifiers (purportedly to help with tooth grinding caused by MDMA) and glow sticks.

While some young people in the nineties were at raves, others were skateboarding (see "Sports and Fashion"), a sport which moved from skateparks in the seventies and into the streets by the nineties. Skateboarders initially wore baggy pants made popular by hip-hop, but distanced themselves from the ravers in the late nineties with slimmer styles. Skate shoes, a necessity for the sport, caught on in the mainstream, with brands like Etnies becoming

a high-school staple. By the early twenty-first century, skateboarding's slacker-cool style was distinct enough for skate culture magazines such as *Color* to run compelling fashion stories, while Supreme transcended being just skate clothing to become one of the most hyped streetwear brands.

The twenty-first century saw the continuation of a lot of subcultures (hip-hop, skate, and goth are still going strong), as well as the proliferation of some new ones. Steampunk is a particularly odd example; at once history- and technology-obsessed, steampunks live in a quaint fantasy world that mixes modern gadgets with nineteenth and early twentieth-century style. Steampunks buy leather cases for their iPhones, and wear Edwardian waistcoats and bowties, or corseted dresses. With its quirky appeal and geeky fanbase, steampunk has inspired a raft of how-to books and provoked concerned online speculation about whether it's set to invade mainstream fashion; meanwhile, it's tough to determine whether

above — Abrasive and hard-edged, punk's sound and aesthetic were rooted in antiestablishment thinking. Shown here, punks in 1980 London stick it to the man with some anarchy graffiti.

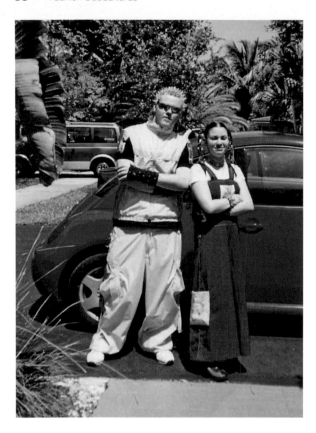

the looks on the runways of designers like Prada, Louis Vuitton, and Alexander McQueen are steampunk inspired, or whether the influence is simply history.

The twenty-first century is also responsible for what is possibly the most reviled subculture ever: hipsters. Obsessed with authenticity, the stereotypical hipster denies being a hipster while simultaneously trying very hard to be cool. A lot of this is simple fashion posing: hipsters are notorious for their skinny jeans, their plaid shirts, their thick plastic glasses, their leather shoes, their handmade or vintage finds. The look easily made its way into the mainstream, and by the second decade of the twenty-first century commentators were laying flowers on the hipster's gravestone—but with a subculture that denies its own existence it's tough to tell whether it's dead, or faking it.

Which brings us back to the Met Ball. It's a sure sign that a subculture has ceased to really be "sub" when its styles have migrated seamlessly into the mainstream ("hipster" being a case in point). But

some subcultures continue on the fringes after their heyday, clinging to their original purpose or finding a new one. Punk may be one of those: with its political insinuations, punk style has been adopted by contemporary antiauthoritarian groups, including Pussy Riot, the radical female performance artists who protest Vladimir Putin's repressive policies. So maybe punk is not dead after all—which would explain why the rich, famous patrons of the Met Ball had such a hard time transforming its subcultural style into red-carpet photo ops.

above — With their oversized clothes, pigtails, and rainbow accessories, candy ravers brought an unironic, childlike sense of fun to the all-night party scene of the 1990s.

right — What's authentic? Hipsters (like this couple in Brick Lane in 2009) spend a lot of time in pursuit of an effortless cool.

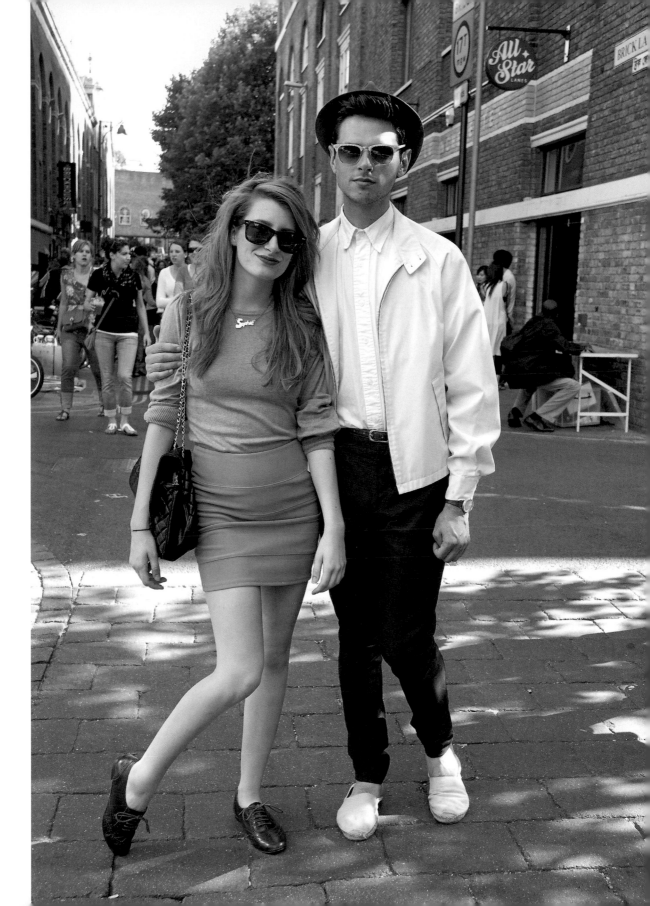

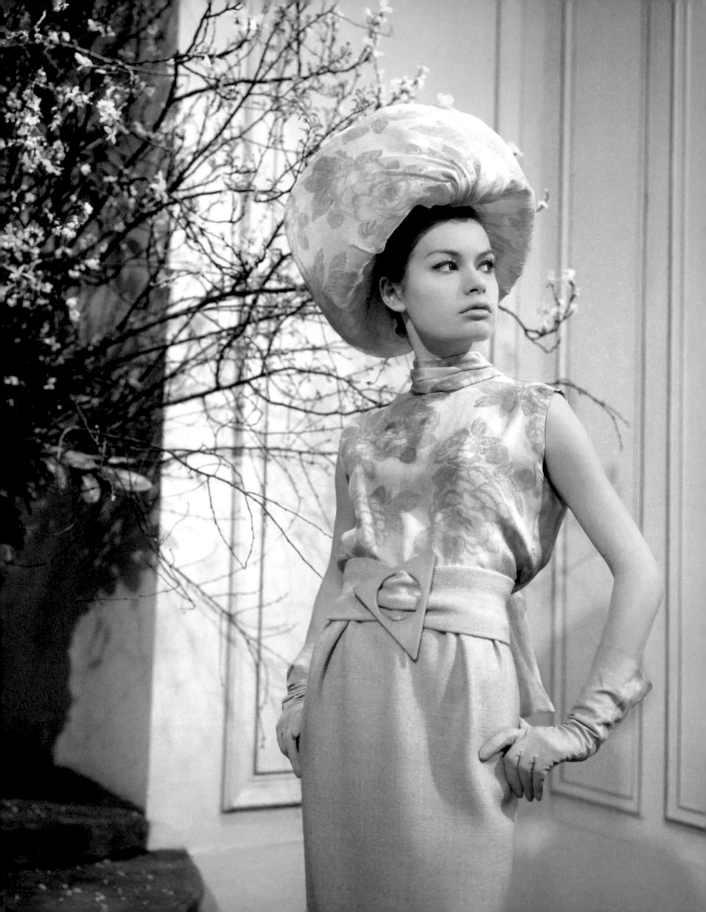

Ready-to-Wear and Mass Fashion

In most people's closets, you'll find rows of shirts and pants and dresses with little tags inside that, in addition to a brand name, say something like "Medium" or "6" or another familiar size: this is ready-to-wear. Defined as clothing in standard sizes, manufactured en masse, and sold from a store literally ready to wear without any modifications, ready-to-wear (or prêt-à-porter in French) has existed in some form for thousands of years; there are records of such clothing being sold in ancient Babylonia. But within fashion, ready-to-wear usually refers to trendy clothing made by high-end designers, produced for purchase at stores. Ready-to-wear debuts each season at fashion weeks in cities like Paris and New York, and in casual conversation it's often confused with couture, the extremely expensive made-to-measure clothing that dominated high-end fashion in the early part of the twentieth century (see "Couture"). But in the mid-twentieth century, the focus of fashion designers shifted from couture to ready-to-wear, and ever since, fashion has been a lot more mass, and a lot less exclusive.

Couturiers as far back as Vionnet and Paul Poiret dabbled with ready-to-wear, but usually out of desperation, and often to the disgust of the fashion industry. In Poiret's case, he designed a ready-to-wear collection for Printemps, the French department store, when his own business was in tatters in 1933. Later on, Jacques Fath experimented with ready-to-wear for both the American and French markets in the late forties and fifties—very unusual at the time. Nobody really embraced ready-to-wear until the demands of the burgeoning youth culture of the sixties (see "Fashion Subcultures") presented the need for more affordable (and more youthful) clothing.

The first couturier to really throw himself into ready-to-wear was Pierre Cardin. He began his couture business in 1950 (with his first collection in 1953), and then launched his ready-to-wear collection in Printemps in 1959. Immediately, he was kicked out of the Chambre syndicale de la haute couture, the organization that regulated couture, but that didn't stop him. He launched his men's ready-to-wear line in 1961, and though he'd been reinstated in the Chambre syndicale, he rebelliously withdrew of his own accord in 1966.

left — Despite slaps on the wrist from the organization regulating couture, Pierre Cardin openly pursued the youth-oriented ready-to-wear market. Shown here is a piece from his Spring/Summer 1962 collection.

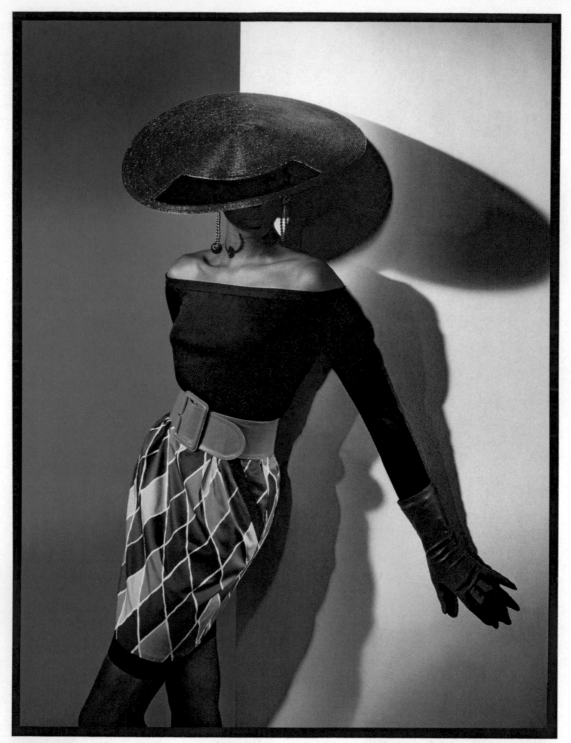

SAINT LAURENT
rive gauche

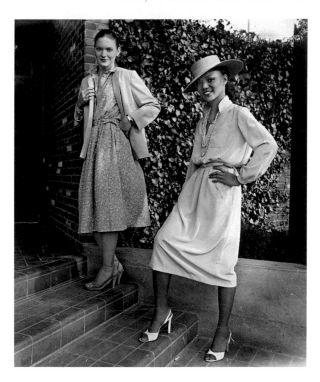

The idea of ready-to-wear being a step in the wrong direction came to an abrupt end when the daring, youthful couturier Yves Saint Laurent opened his dedicated ready-to-wear shop, Rive Gauche, in Paris in 1966, quickly followed by another location in London in 1969. Rive Gauche was insanely popular, a veritable fashion sensation. Rather than presenting ready-to-wear as a spinoff of couture, or derivative of it, it became Saint Laurent's cause célèbre. In the aftermath of his couture collection in 1971, which flopped, he declared that he intended to use ready-to-wear as his primary fashion platform, rather than couture. With its name taken from the Left Bank, Paris's center of bohemian life, Rive Gauche

diametrically opposed the stuffiness of the traditional couture houses (which were located on the Right Bank), in perfect timing with youth culture's fashion needs.

After Saint Laurent's revolutionary move, fashion's snooty attitude toward ready-to-wear changed; not only did it become the norm for couture designers to maintain ready-to-wear lines to diversify their revenue streams, but, in fact, ready-to-wear became the primary vehicle through which designers could show their stuff. By 1973, Pierre Bergé—Saint Laurent's partner in both life and business—formed the Chambre syndicale du prêt-à-porter des couturiers et des créateurs de mode to regulate the now thriving ready-to-wear industry.

The move toward mass-producing luxury fashion went even further in the seventies and eighties, when licensing deals exploded. In licensing, a designer would sell the rights to use their name to a secondary producer, allowing them to slap the designer's brand onto whatever goods they were selling: T-shirts, watches, luggage, you name it. One of the pioneers of ready-to-wear, Pierre Cardin, became particularly known for his licensing deals.

left — Anything but gauche, Yves Saint Laurent's Rive Gauche (advertised here in 1986–87) elevated ready-to-wear to the height of cool.

above — Halston's ready-to-wear brought a little 1970s disco chic to off-the-rack fashion (the models shown wear a Liberty design on the left, and Halston on the right, in 1972).

He happily licensed his name to companies to produce all manner of goods: handbags, home decor, watches, and more. By the millennium, he had hundreds of licensing agreements. Pierre Cardin goods were everywhere, blanketing the retail environment, and selling for very low prices. Unsurprisingly, this massively diluted his brand image and cheapened the Pierre Cardin name. Of course, not every designer was as promiscuous with licensing, and many found it to be an excellent strategy for widening the appeal of their brand.

One of the stars of seventies fashion, Roy Halston Frowick (who designed as Halston), also brought some interesting changes to the ready-to-wear industry. A darling of the New York fashion scene in the seventies, Halston became known equally for his minimalist looks (particularly his shirtdresses and slinky garments made from his favorite material, Ultrasuede) and, later, for his over-the-top cocaine-and-Quaaludes party lifestyle. He began designing hats in 1958, created his first clothing collection for Bergdorf Goodman in 1966, and had his own multi-story boutique by 1972. But by the eighties, Halston's social escapades had taken their toll on his business, and he had to do something. In 1982, he made a monumental decision that today is practically banal, but in the eighties was sacrilege: he signed a deal with J. C. Penney to create a mass fashion line, in the spirit of today's designer collaborations. Sadly, for Halston, the industry wasn't ready for this particular innovation. His ready-to-wear line was ejected from Bergdorf Goodman, and Halston was done as a fashion designer.

While ready-to-wear originally defined itself as couture's more affordable cousin, it doesn't strive to be down-market; today, ready-to-wear's appeal lies in the idea that it makes luxury available to the average person. Armani, the keystone of Italian ready-to-wear, is a prime example of ready-to-wear and mass fashion that fastidiously maintained an aura of

right — Fashion's blue period began in 1978, when Calvin Klein ushered in the era of luxury jeans (worn here by Brooke Shields in a 1980 advertisement).

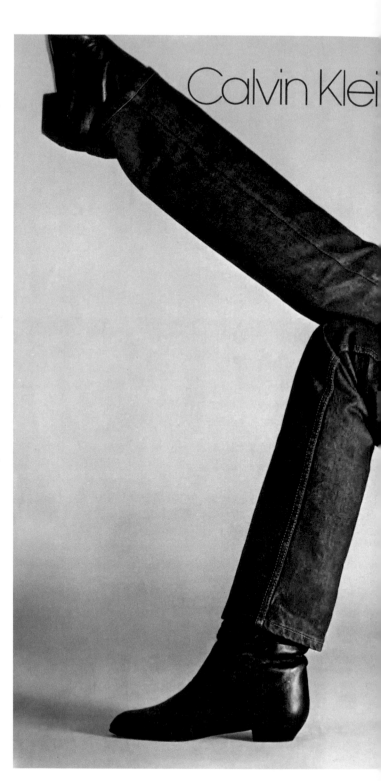

eans

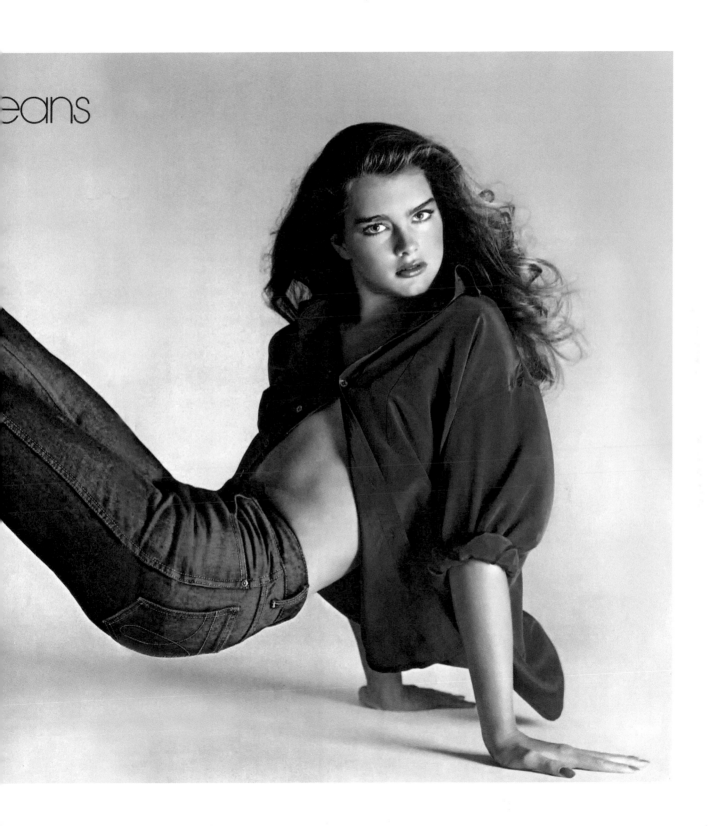

luxury. Giorgio Armani came up with an interesting arrangement where he personally supervised the manufacture, in a factory setting, of his ready-to-wear, thus ensuring its quality. He became famous for his clean lines and unstructured garments, in particular his unlined jackets, in the late seventies and early eighties.

The eighties and nineties were boom time for ready-to-wear, as the industry became more vertically integrated and brands united under larger conglomerates. Luxury jeans became a staple of high-end fashion in the eighties after Calvin Klein showed jeans in his ready-to-wear show in 1976, and "lifestyle branding" came to the fore via Ralph Lauren's aggressive portrayal of American life through his massively successful, preppy ready-to-wear collections.

By the new millennium, fashion was ready to go even more mass, this time via designer collaborations, where a major designer would pair with a mass fashion chain (Halston was way ahead of his time). One of the first entries into the designer collaboration game was Isaac Mizrahi for Target in 2002. He was followed quickly in 2004 by the shape-shifting Karl Lagerfeld, who had designed successfully for multiple houses over his career, including Balmain, Patou, Chloé, and Fendi, but whose name at that point was primarily tied to his role as the artistic director (and savior) of Chanel. No stranger to ready-to-wear, Lagerfeld had also run his own eponymous ready-to-wear line. It may seem a peculiar choice for Lagerfeld to align himself with H&M, the massive Swedish chain known for ultra-cheap (but trendy) attire—quintessential mall fashion. However, going mass was Lagerfeld's explicit

aim, and he later expressed regret that H&M produced his looks in such limited quantities.

After the Lagerfeld x H&M collection, high/low designer/retail collaborations became an industry obsession. At H&M, collaborators included Stella McCartney, Comme des Garçons, Lanvin—and, to everybody's amazement, Versace. The Versace collection became a hot-ticket item, appearing on veritable fashion icons like Kanye West and Anna Dello Russo—people who could afford the real thing rather than the so-called masstige version. Suddenly, what was available to the masses was what was coveted, and lining up for the launch of an H&M collection (and later seeing it on eBay, with jacked-up prices) became normal. Owning one of these pieces spoke less to an individual's net worth than to their tenacity to suffer in a line overnight for a limited-edition mass-fashion item. Through these sought-after collaborations, large, mass-produced fashion lines have managed to acquire an air of exclusivity. It's tough to say whether this sort of thing is sustainable, or whether, as happened with Pierre Cardin and Halston, designer label mass fashion will architect its own demise with its ready availability. But those lines in front of H&M in cities around the globe have proven one thing for certain: people are hungry for designer fashion and the status that comes with it, whatever the cost.

right — Karl Lagerfeld looms large over fashion, even more so after his collaborations with mass-fashion retailer H&M. Here he is pictured in a campaign ad on a billboard in central Berlin alongside model Erin Wasson in 2004.

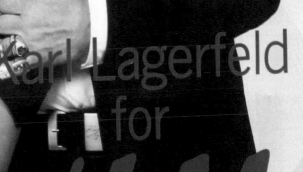

Feminism and Fashion

In May 2013, venerable fashion designer Miuccia Prada confessed to the *New York Times' T Magazine*, "When I started [in the seventies], fashion was the worst place to be if you were a leftist feminist. It was horrid. I had a prejudice, yes, I always had a problem with it." It's an unfortunate truth: feminism and fashion have not always been friends. Their relationship has suffered due to two opposing ideas: that fashion is a powerful tool women can use to forge identity and influence others, or that fashion is a force that oppresses women. There may, in fact, be a little truth in both. Though fashion has been used by women to achieve power and influence for many years (Marie Antoinette is a particularly notable example; see "Royal Fashion"), feminism has long regarded this as playing by patriarchy's rules. The feminist movement, which aims for real equality between the sexes rather than fleeting power within a male-dominated culture, didn't take root until the mid-nineteenth century. And the movement's most prominent early leaders, part of what is now called feminism's First Wave,

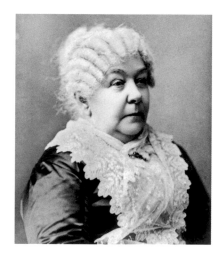

were Susan B. Anthony and Elizabeth Cady Stanton, Puritans who disapproved of fashionable dress. In fact, at the 1852 Women's Convention, Elizabeth Stanton opposed the leadership bid of a devoted feminist, Elizabeth Oakes Smith, based on her stylish attire. Cady Stanton's attitude has held throughout much of feminism's history: it is impossible to be both fashionable and a feminist.

At the time of feminism's birth, women's clothing was far more about form than function. Tightly laced corsets and heavy skirts may have cut a dramatic

above — No fan of fashion, Elizabeth Cady Stanton (shown here in 1910) was a pivotal figure in the suffrage movement.

right — With her garçonne look, Chanel (photographed here in 1936) popularized mannish fashion that allowed women the freedom to really move.

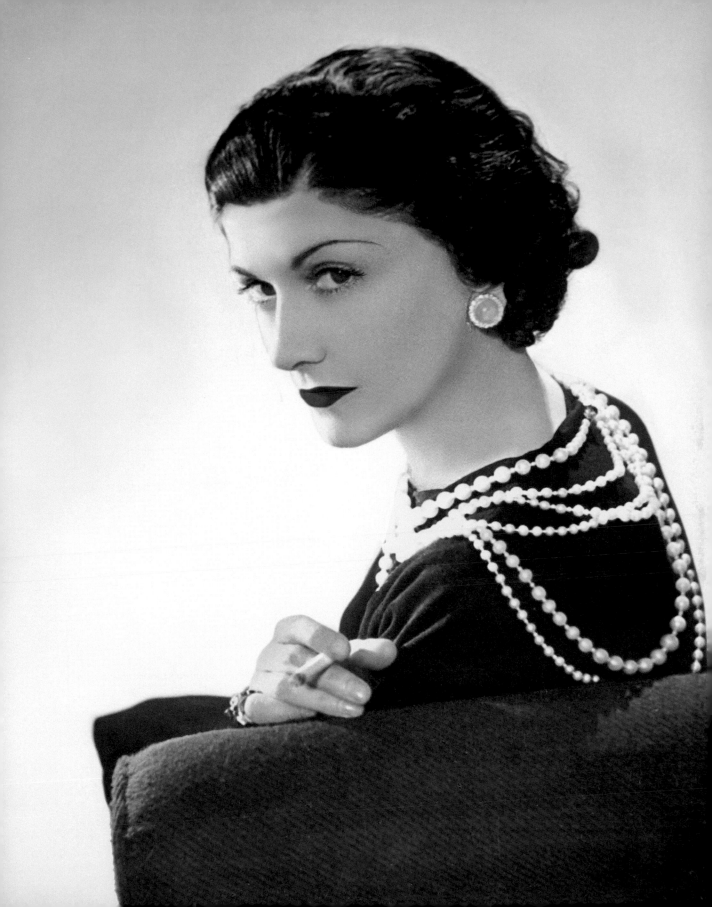

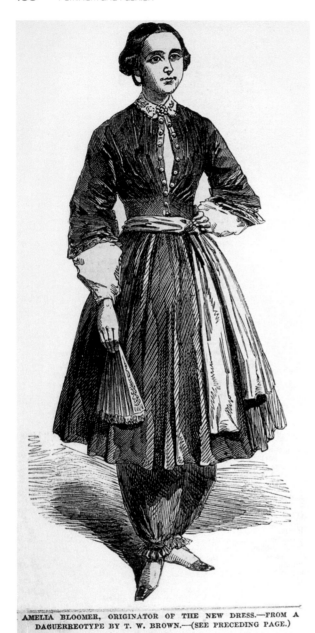

AMELIA BLOOMER, ORIGINATOR OF THE NEW DRESS.—FROM A DAGUERREOTYPE BY T. W. BROWN.—(SEE PRECEDING PAGE.)

left — Bloomin' awesome: Amelia Bloomer started a small fashion craze in 1851 when she slipped on a pair of ankle-tapered pants.

right — Tomboyish Coco Chanel made the clothes that she wanted to wear; here she models one of her fashionable tailored suits in 1929.

figure, but they were uncomfortable, difficult to move about in, and raised health concerns. It is no surprise, then, that one of feminism's most visible early moves was a radical fashion statement: bloomers. In 1851, Amelia Bloomer, who edited a journal devoted to temperance and women's rights called *The Lily*, was shown an outfit by Elizabeth Cady Stanton: a dress with trousers underneath, similar to what Turkish women wore. Bloomer adopted it, wrote about it in

The Lily, and started a minor fashion craze. The billowing, ankle-tapered trousers, named "bloomers" due to Amelia's influence, even made it into *Harper's Monthly*. But it wasn't all positive attention. Bloomers were also the subject of much ridicule, including satire in *Punch*. Whether due to mockery or fading interest, the trend died quickly. Nevertheless, bloomers are notable as Western women's first experiment with trousers.

Though they did not identify as feminists, two couturiers from the twentieth century deserve special mention for the progress they brought to women's attire. The first of these is Madeleine Vionnet. At the time Vionnet was designing, women's clothing was still constrictive; even Paul Poiret, much lauded for emancipating the female figure, used corsets, albeit looser ones. Vionnet threw all that away, relying on the natural curves of women's bodies. Her designs utilized draping and—her great contribution to couture—the bias cut, which made her dresses cling to the body in an appealing way. Vionnet's designs were radical, but they were also the first triumph of the female figure in modern fashion.

Active at the same time as Vionnet, Coco Chanel revolutionized couture by popularizing masculine-inspired fashion for women—blazers, sweaters, jersey suits. Understated and well tailored, these

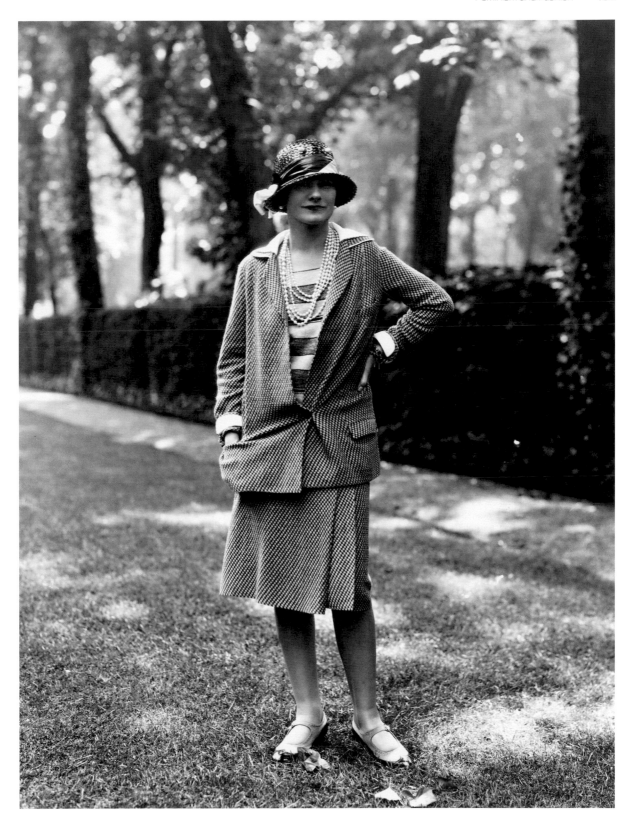

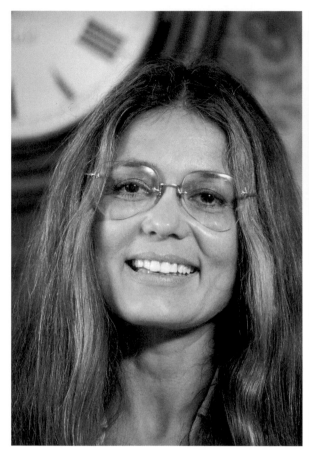

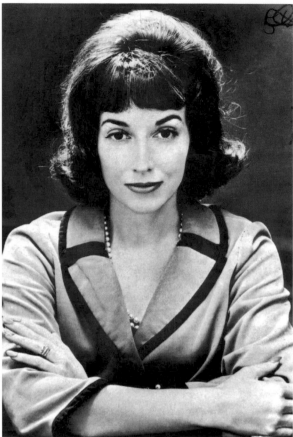

were clothes that brought a new meaning to chic, but at the same time were highly versatile and allowed women to live an active life while remaining stylish.

Of course, women's newly vigorous lifestyles of the time were indebted to both the mobilization of women into the workforce during World War I as well as the triumphs of the feminist movement. By the twenties, when Chanel and Vionnet's designs were in vogue, the United States, the United Kingdom, and most other Western countries had granted women the right to vote, and the first wave of feminism had achieved its primary goal.

After World War II, society's mood became a lot more conservative: the perfect environment for Christian Dior's ultrafeminine New Look to thrive. Launching to great acclaim in 1947, the New Look brought hourglass curves back into fashion, with full skirts and a small waist made possible by a modified

corset called a "waist cincher." The look horrified Coco Chanel so much that she burst out of retirement in 1954, aged seventy-one, to bring practical clothing back to women again.

Postwar domesticity also prompted another reaction: Second Wave feminism, spurred by Betty Friedan's seminal 1963 book *The Feminine Mystique*, which held up the example of the bored, miserable housewife as an argument that women were not

above left — As feminism's reluctant cover girl, Gloria Steinem's obvious style at times earned her criticism. She is shown here in 1974 wearing her trademark aviator glasses.

above right — Her va-va-voom vixens and please-your-man tactics may seem dated today, but in 1963 self-identified feminist Helen Gurley Brown was focused on women getting ahead.

destined to find happiness solely through maintaining a household. And so Second Wave feminism defined its aim: equality for women in the workplace. The Second Wave coexisted with the sexual revolution, symbolized by the Pill and the miniskirt, though the latter was never really embraced as a feminist symbol.

Unlike earlier feminists, those of the seventies were photographed for mainstream magazines and featured on television. And feminism found itself a very fashionable figurehead for those purposes: Gloria Steinem. Already well-known for her magazine writing—she'd even been featured in a 1965 *Newsweek* profile that declared her "the thinking man's Jean Shrimpton"—Steinem was unhappy with the topics that editors frequently pushed her toward beauty and fashion. She was more interested in politics. In 1968, she found feminism, and by 1972 she launched *Ms.* magazine to provide a serious, non-fluffy alternative to the women's magazines at the time. Despite her dismissive attitude toward fashion, she was (and still is) adept at managing her public image, and clearly cultivated a look. Her hip-huggers, blond-streaked hair, and aviator sunglasses became a signature style that was widely imitated. She was feminism's cover girl—which, despite bringing more attention to the feminist movement, earned her harsh criticism, another instance of friction between feminism and fashion. Women's workplace aspirations and the fashions that came with them also changed the environment at fashion magazines, most dramatically at *Vogue*, where the eccentric visionary Diana Vreeland was ousted in favor of beige-loving Grace Mirabella in 1971 (see "Fashion Magazines"). Mirabella's goal was to tailor the magazine to the needs of the working woman. She featured the sort of clothing that would be at home in an office—smart and affordable, sometimes power-suited. It many ways, it was the physical manifestation of Second Wave feminism, but many mourned the loss of artistic verve in the magazine.

At the other end of the spectrum was Helen Gurley Brown, author of the upwardly mobile siren bible *Sex and the Single Girl* and infamous editor of *Cosmopolitan*. Gurley Brown self-identified as a feminist—unsurprising, given that her ideas were all about women succeeding in the workplace. Nonetheless, she was widely derided by feminists at the time, largely because of the way she advocated for sex as both a pleasurable pastime and a tool for getting ahead. And while it wasn't a fashion magazine per se, *Cosmo*'s man-pleasing style had a lasting impact on women's attitudes toward dressing. It was all about big hair and big cleavage and figure-hugging attire. *Cosmo*'s full-throttle vixens later became a caricature of female sexuality, but at the time they were revolutionary.

Being fashionable, sexy, or image-conscious wasn't really accepted by feminism until the Third Wave of the early nineties, which was largely a reaction against the failures of the Second Wave to embrace

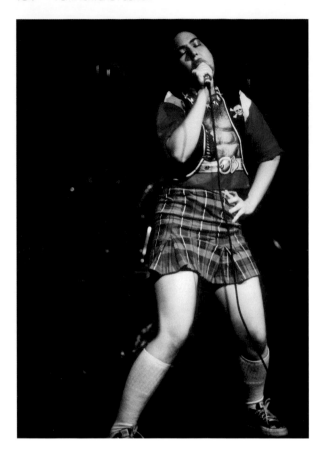

left — Unabashedly flaunting her sexuality, Bikini Kill's Kathleen Hanna (performing here in 1994) was the embodiment of riot grrrl's sex-positive Third Wave feminism.

the plurality of female experience—including the desire to dress up. One of the Third Wave's manifestations was riot grrrl, a DIY cultural movement centered on female-fronted music and zines. Riot grrrl was influenced by punk (see "Fashion and Music"), but its fashion was openly girly and sexually aggressive, with Bikini Kill's Kathleen Hanna wearing "slutty" outfits as a kind of protest against their perceived sluttiness. One of riot grrrl's descendants, oddly, was "Girl Power," a somewhat vacuous statement of female empowerment popularized by British pop group the Spice Girls, mostly useful as a slogan on T-shirts. Around the same time, in the eighties and nineties, Madonna was defiantly using highly sexualized fashion (like the cone bra designed by Jean Paul Gaultier) to define her image, which caused some to point to her as the embodiment of the Third Wave.

In the present day, it doesn't draw gasps when feminists wear fashionable clothes. And yet, the question of whether fashion and feminism can coexist is still

frequently asked—after all, the feminist media's acknowledgement that fashion matters to women, and that this might be okay, is new. For example, Gawker Media property *Jezebel*, arguably the web's most popular feminist publication, regularly covers fashion (trends, labels, and icons) in its "Rag Trade" column, while one of the web's most popular fashion bloggers, Tavi (see "Fashion and the Internet"), uses her teen style and culture website *Rookie* as a platform to instill her nascent feminism into a young audience. Meanwhile, fashion blog *Man Repeller* puts a different spin on fashion: rather than a tool to beguile men, fashion's weirder and more experimental silhouettes often turn them off, as the title of the blog suggests. A far cry from the idea that fashion oppresses women, it celebrates the idea that women are dressing up for each other, and for themselves. As Third Wave feminism awkwardly embraces fashion, it is unclear where this relationship is headed. But it's nice to know that as women work it out, they can choose to put on some stylish clothes—or not. It's all up to them.

right — She found her voice in fashion, but blogger Tavi Gevinson (shown here in 2013) uses her stylish website for teen girls, *Rookie*, to start conversations about feminism.

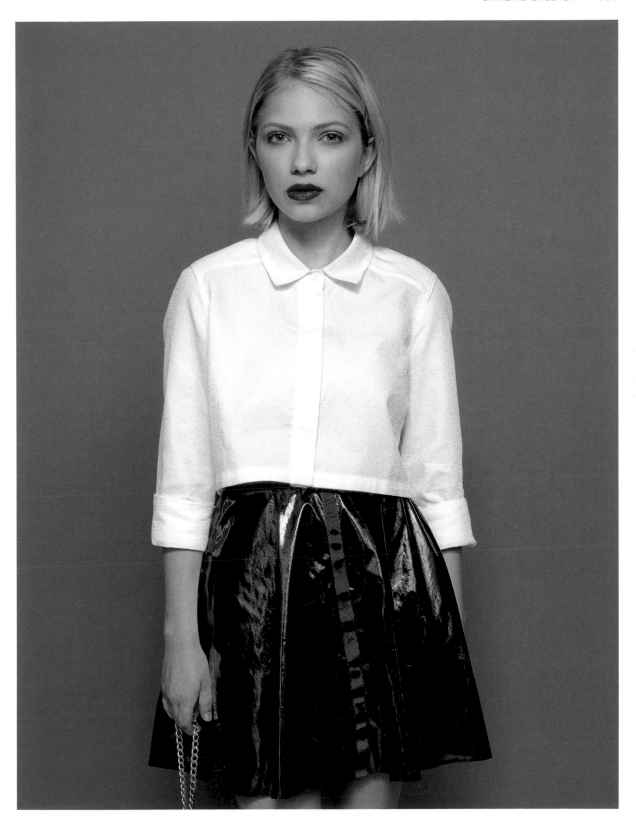

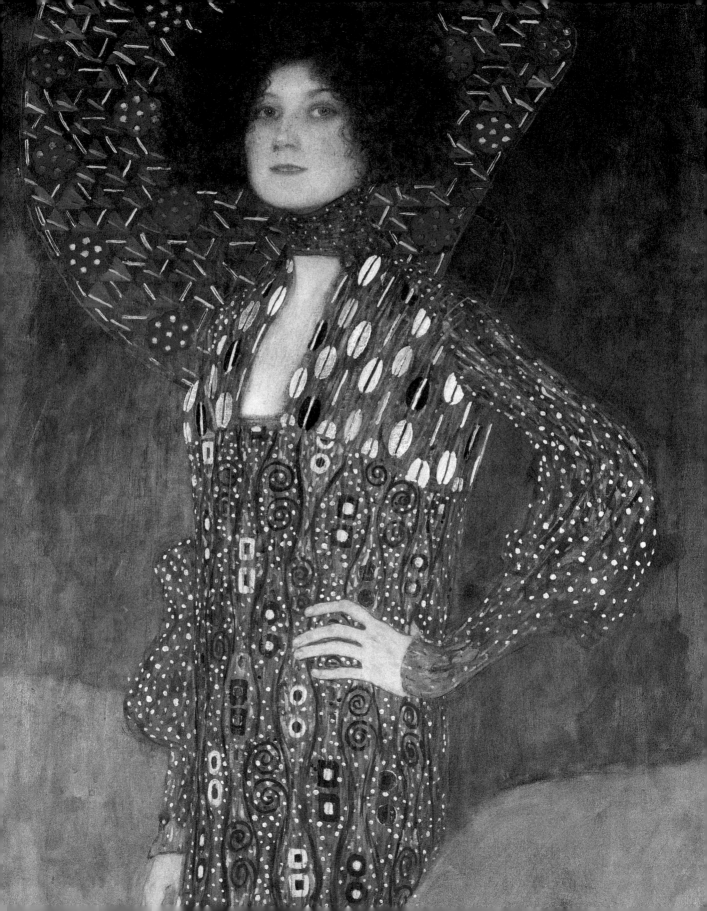

Fashion and Art

The day it opened to the public in 2011, the line for *Alexander McQueen: Savage Beauty*, the rebellious British designer's retrospective exhibit at New York's Metropolitan Museum of Art, stretched for two city blocks. Over its run, the show broke attendance records, and fans of McQueen's emotional, elaborate, and theatrical fashions couldn't stop talking about the show. It's rare for an exhibition at an art museum to spark this kind of excitement, but McQueen inspired a devoted fandom not seen by many contemporary artists. This, of course, raises the question: Is fashion art?

Modern audiences seem to think so, but there's no critical agreement on whether fashion, which is tied up in commerce and human vanity, can match the aesthetic purity and conceptual complexity of "real" art. Nonetheless, fashion and art share a long history together, cross-pollinating each other along the way, and sometimes cooperating to create beautiful hybrids.

Modern fashion and art both bloomed in the aftermath of the Industrial Revolution, which triggered the rise of a middle class obsessed with the pursuit of individuality and self-expression. The mid-nineteenth century marks the beginning of couture (see "Couture"), whose earliest designers, like Charles Frederick Worth, believed themselves to be artists. Worth studied paintings in the National Gallery in London for fashion inspiration when he was young. By the time he was an established Parisian couturier with devoted clients and a reputation for artistry, he began to dress like an artist, costuming himself in a beret and a cravat.

Worth's attention to art wasn't just a childhood thing; his couture, as well as that of others of the time, took tips from the Art Nouveau movement, which infused most of the decorative arts at the turn of the century. Inspired by nature, Art Nouveau was known for its curvaceous vines and serpentine florals, which took shape in patterning: embroidery, appliqué, and lace motifs swirled prettily around the era's couture dresses.

Worth wasn't alone in considering himself an artist; the rebellious couturier Paul Poiret, who dominated Parisian fashion in the early twentieth century, also had artistic pretensions. As a teenager he spent much time in the Louvre seeking inspiration for his fashion sketches, and after his later successes in couture (and the money that came with it) he

left —Designer, businesswoman, and Gustav Klimt's life partner, Emilie Flöge modeled many of Klimt's radical dress designs in his paintings (as here, in 1902).

became a well-known art collector. Poiret was particularly fond of Fauve paintings, a style that used bright colors and strong brushstrokes, whose principal artists were Henri Matisse and André Derain. Inspired by these paintings, Poiret began using vivid colors in his designs: pinks, blues, purples, golds, and greens. This predated the arrival of the Ballets Russes in Paris, which sparked a tidal wave of interest in rich colors and Eastern fashions—Poiret was the trendsetter, due to the influence of art. His Orientalist designs are often cited as an example of Art Deco in fashion.

Though couture borrowed from art, many artists between the turn of the century and the middle of the century worked in opposition to the trends of the time. One of the most famous artists to cross the boundary between art and fashion was Gustav Klimt, the most prominent member of the Viennese Secession movement. The Secessionists believed that all arts, including the "minor" arts such as fashion, were important, and so applied themselves to dress. As well as designing robes for himself, Klimt made dresses for his life partner Emilie Flöge, who ran a fashion boutique in Vienna. Klimt's dresses flew in the face of couture: they were loose, exotic, patterned garments, the opposite of a fitted gown. Meanwhile, in Italy, the Futurist art movement had

its sights on reforming every aspect of life to make it more modern, including fashion. Futurists believed that when it came to artistic value, fashion was on a par with painting, and they issued manifestos to outline their approach to modernizing dress. Among the Futurists, the first to design fashion was Giacomo Balla, in 1912. He designed for both men and women, and his creations utilized asymmetrical cuts and color blocks to create a feeling of movement. Some of his fashions also featured "modifiers," colored patches that could be fixed anywhere on a garment; the designs of the Futurists are sometimes cited as an influence on people like Paul Poiret, as well as another artist, Sonia Delaunay.

Sonia Delaunay's forays into fashion competed somewhat with the Futurists. An artist herself, Delaunay often receives credit for bringing Cubist influence to fashion. She and her husband, Robert Delaunay, experimented with a form called "simultaneous painting," featuring blocks of contrasting

right — With his self-image as an artist, it's no surprise that Charles Frederick Worth took inspiration from art; this evening dress from 1893 features Art Nouveau detailing.

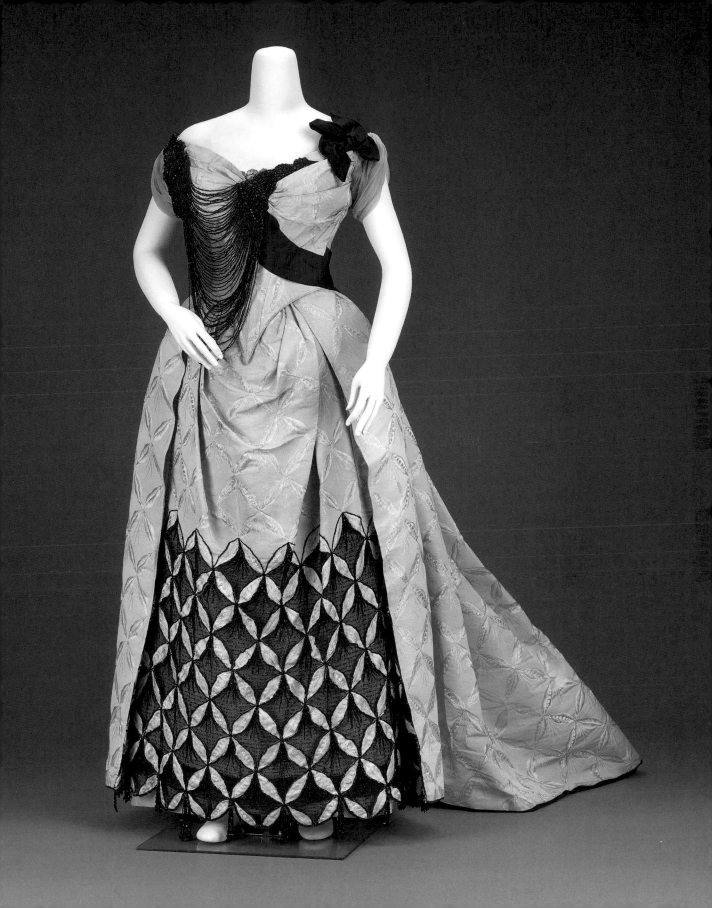

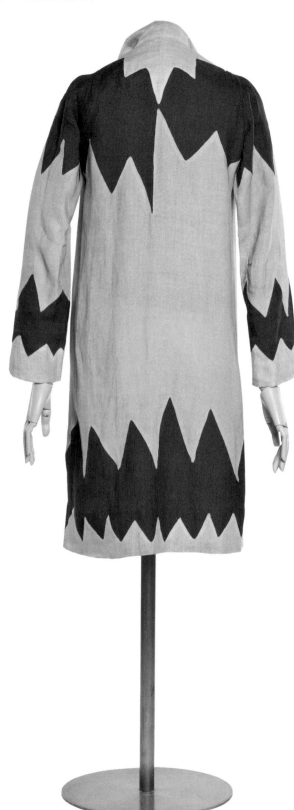

color. She began designing clothes in 1913, debuting them among the Parisian avant-garde to much effect (including a write-up from Guillaume Apollinaire). Delaunay championed a more creative style of dressing, moving away from what she saw as the strict confines of couture: her aims were not to supplement fashion, but to revolutionize it. By 1927, she was so known for her clothing that she gave a lecture at the Sorbonne titled "The Influence of Painting on Fashion."

Though couture borrowed from art and art rebelled against couture, it wasn't long before the two collaborated. The outrageously provocative couturier Elsa Schiaparelli finally brought artists and couturiers into creative union in the thirties. Schiaparelli always aimed to shock, and for her the weird and dreamlike creations of the Surrealists were serious fashion fodder. She integrated Surrealism into fashion, but with the explicit involvement of the artists themselves. Her work with Salvador Dalí is her most famous; among her collaborations with him are a coat inspired by his woman made of drawers, and

left — Sonia Delaunay's Cubist clothing gave her an edge within the Parisian avant-garde. Shown here is one of her coat designs of 1925.

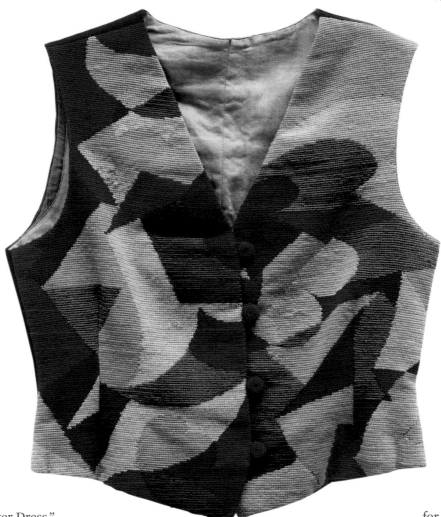

her "Lobster Dress,"
featuring a crustacean
painted by Dalí onto the skirt. Her
1937 work with Jean Cocteau also turned heads: an
embroidered coat where the outlines of two kissing
women form an optical illusion of a vase with flowers.
One of fashion's traits sometimes blamed as an
impediment to its artistic relevance is its commercialism. But in the seventies, that wasn't much of an
issue for Andy Warhol, whose Pop Art was openly
inspired by commercialism and celebrity. Warhol's
Factory, the New York studio and gathering space

above —Rooted in a philosophy of modernization, Futurist
fashion like that made by Giacomo Balla featured asymmetrical shapes and a revolutionary sense of movement. Shown
here is his "futuristic vest" of 1924–25.

for his circle of
creatives, was a petri
dish for art and style, and many
of the people who hung around the Factory, such
as Edie Sedgwick, became fashion icons. There was
an incestuous relationship between the Factory and
Paraphernalia, Betsey Johnson's shop; the Velvet
Underground performed there, and Betsey Johnson
married John Cale, one of the members of the band.
Soon, Edie Sedgwick became a Paraphernalia model.
Warhol's ties to the fashion world extended outside
the Factory, too. He experimented with silkscreen-
ing on paper dresses, which were popular in the sixties, and his friend Halston designed clothing using
Warhol flower prints. Warhol himself was highly
interested in using clothing as part of his character;
he dressed impeccably and swannishly, and even
spent some time as a runway model. After his death,
his wardrobe was used as an exhibition at the Andy

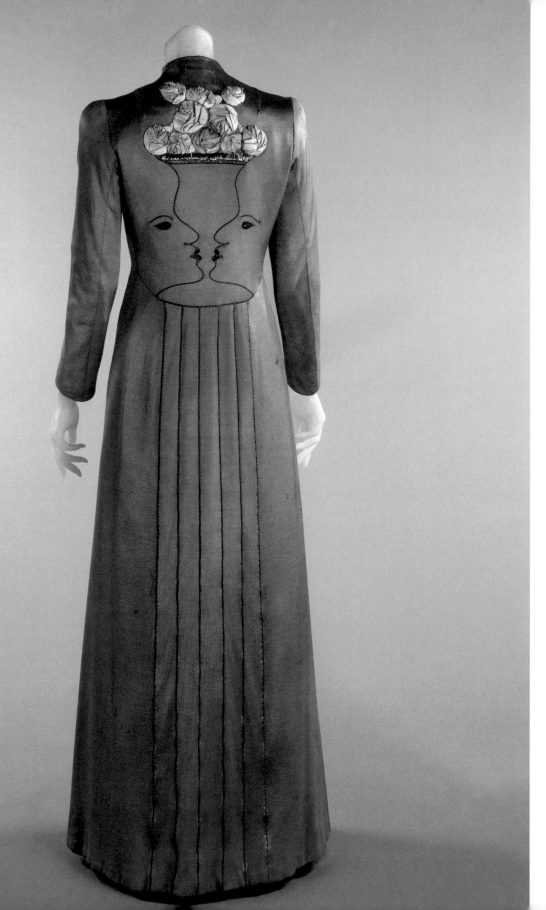

Warhol Museum. Warhol's influence in fashion had longevity, and his prints remain a heavily used motif today.

The late-sixties art world was also the source of one of modern fashion's most influential themes: minimalism. Originally seen in the work of artists like Donald Judd and Agnes Martin, its simplicity was soon integrated into fashion design (or, some argue, its terms were applied to existing design trends). Sixties fashion became fascinated by straight edges and clean lines; Yves Saint Laurent's "Mondrian" dress, even as it referenced an earlier art movement with its print, was an excellent example of the sixties minimalist form. For fashion writers, minimalism

left — Artist/designer collaborations were the brainchild of edgy couturier Elsa Schiaparelli, who regularly worked with high-profile artists like Jean Cocteau; she created this eye-catching surrealist coat with him in 1937.

above — The essence of sleek modernism, Yves Saint Laurent's 1965 collection was inspired by Dutch artist Piet Mondrian; his iconic "Mondrian" dress has been repeated and copied in designs ever since. Shown here is a version from YSL's 2002 collection.

was a handy reference. And it has remained one up to the present day; in the nineties, minimalism staged a comeback with the sleek forms of Marc Jacobs and Calvin Klein.

By the eighties, art was coming in from the streets with graffiti's growing artistic legitimacy; the most notable fashion designer to harness this chaotic form was Stephen Sprouse. Sprouse's garments were sophisticated, brightly colored, and energetic, and he adorned many of them with his own graffiti. He also successfully collaborated with graffiti artist Keith Haring to create prints for his Fall 1988 collection. Though his original line was shuttered due to financial difficulties, Spouse was critically successful and his designs maintained a cult appeal. After Sprouse's 2004 death, Marc Jacobs used the designer's 1987

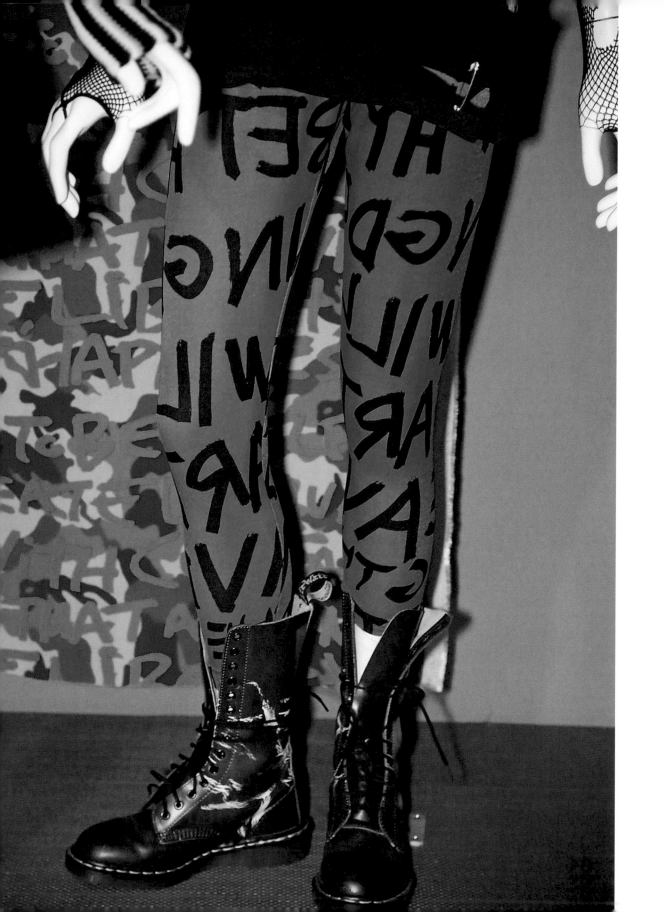

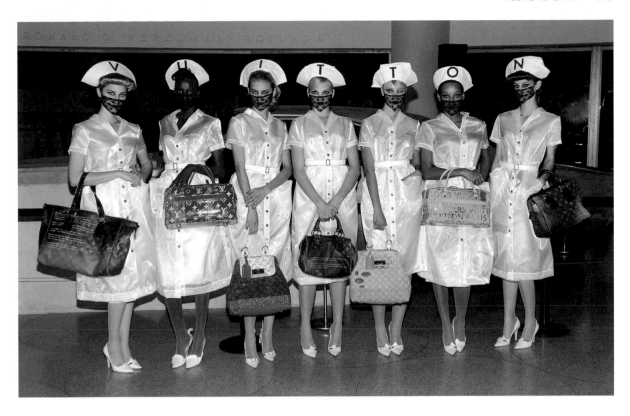

prints for his Louis Vuitton collections in 2006–08. Artist collaborations with major brands have become an important theme in modern fashion; they're a way for artists to profit off fashion, and for designer labels to maintain an edge. Many of the most interesting collaborations have been under Marc Jacobs's watch at Louis Vuitton. One of Vuitton's most notable collaborations was with Takashi Murakami, who painted his artwork over the brand's monogrammed bags in 2007. The year 2008 saw LV collaborate with Richard Prince, who also spray-painted Vuitton bags; the brand even made

left — High fashion got some downtown edge with Stephen Sprouse's graffiti-adorned collections in the early 1980s. Shown here are leggings from his 1985 collection.

above — Art infusion: Louis Vuitton regularly collaborates with artists like Richard Prince, whose handbags are shown here in 2007.

a sly nod to his nurse paintings with their runway show, which featured models in see-through nurse attire. Jacobs shows no signs of abandoning collaborations as a strategy: in 2013, Louis Vuitton commissioned street artists Retna, Aiko, and Os Gêmeos to design scarves.

Even as it uses art to stay culturally relevant, early twenty-first-century fashion takes itself ever more seriously as an art form. Alexander McQueen's show at the Met was only one of many displays of designer collections shown in art galleries in recent years. Other examples include Yves Saint Laurent's retrospective, *Yves Saint Laurent Style*, which debuted in 2008 at the Musée des beaux-arts de Montréal, and *The Fashion World of Jean Paul Gaultier*, which opened in Montreal in 2011 and continues to travel. With the jaw-dropping attendance numbers at the McQueen show, fashion in art museums is something we're likely to see more and more. Is it art? That's not a question with an easy answer. But fashion, like art, offers a visual document of the zeitgeist, and for that its place in museums is probably well deserved.

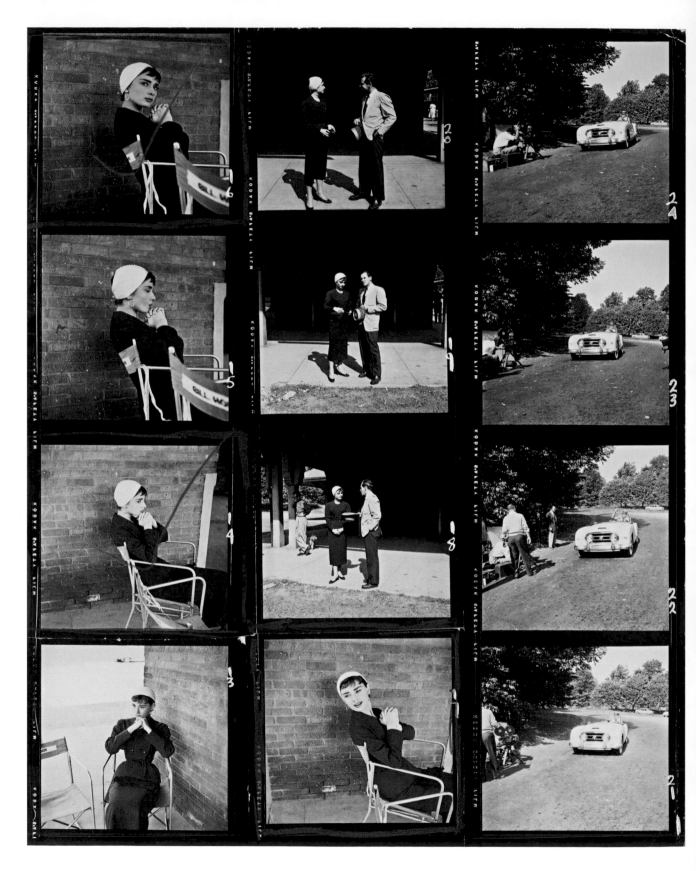

Fashion and Film

When Baz Luhrmann's glitzy, eye-popping version of *The Great Gatsby* hit screens in spring 2013, headlines gasped appreciatively: "Flapper fashions are back!" Beaded dresses and headbands sparkled in magazine spreads, and department stores reported a spike in tuxedo sales for men. No surprise: film is one of the biggest influences on the public's fashion imagination, a lucky privilege it has held for almost a century.

In its early days, on-screen fashion was a disorganized affair. There was no costume department, and actors and actresses were expected to dress themselves. This changed in the twenties with the advent of color film, when studios realized that things looked different on screen, and that a trained eye was necessary to ensure a polished look. Soon all the studios had fully stocked costume departments that designed and sewed costumes for screen productions.

Film's power to shape public taste soon became clear. When Marlene Dietrich donned trousers in the film *Morocco* in 1930—a daring move at the time—it caused a sensation. *It Happened One Night* created an even bigger controversy in 1934, when its star, Clark Gable, took off his shirt to reveal he was wearing nothing underneath but a scandalously bare chest. The sales of undershirts tumbled, and things would never really be the same.

Prior to Hollywood's dominance of popular culture, the biggest influence on fashion was Parisian couturiers (see "Couture"). But since the ascendance of Hollywood and its stars, there's been an ongoing rivalry between fashion designers and costume designers. In the early years of Hollywood, from the twenties through the forties, the two worlds were largely separate, with couturiers reigning in Paris, and costume designers ruling Hollywood. Studios recruited and groomed costume designers, some of them even aspiring couturiers. One of the first was Howard Greer, a designer who began working at Lucile and, after serving in World War II, continued with turns at Paul Poiret and Molyneux, later moving into design for the stage. Due to his background in costume design, he was recruited for Paramount in 1921. Greer was a trailblazer, creating the very first costume design department for Paramount before leaving in 1927 to open his own couture house. Greer's successor was Travis Banton, who

left — The clothes make the lady, as proven by Audrey Hepburn in *Sabrina* (1954), whose titular character dons Givenchy and transforms her life.

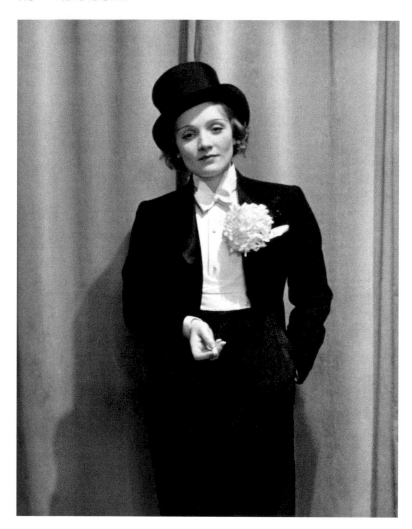

worked as chief designer at Paramount until 1938. Banton designed for many stars, like flapper starlet Clara Bow and vampy Mae West, but he's most notable for his collaborations with Marlene Dietrich. He was largely responsible for her iconoclastic style: it was his idea to put her in trousers, and he designed for her repeatedly over the years.

Hollywood's most celebrated costume designer was, by far, Edith Head. When Banton left Paramount, Head took over from him as chief designer, working there until 1967, when she moved to Universal (she died while in their employment in 1981). Head's design style was restrained, but highly popular, and she became a star favorite. In total, she was nominated for thirty-five Oscars, and won eight—the

record for a woman. Among her achievements, she transformed Dorothy Lamour into a star with her creative costuming (mostly involving a sarong) in *The Jungle Princess*; she also adapted the curves of Dior's New Look to the screen, giving it huge

above — In *Morocco*, Marlene Dietrich drove audiences wild with her transgressive cross-dressing, spurring women to give trousers a try.

right — The grand dame of costume design, Edith Head (shown here in 1955) had a career in Hollywood design departments spanning fifty-seven years.

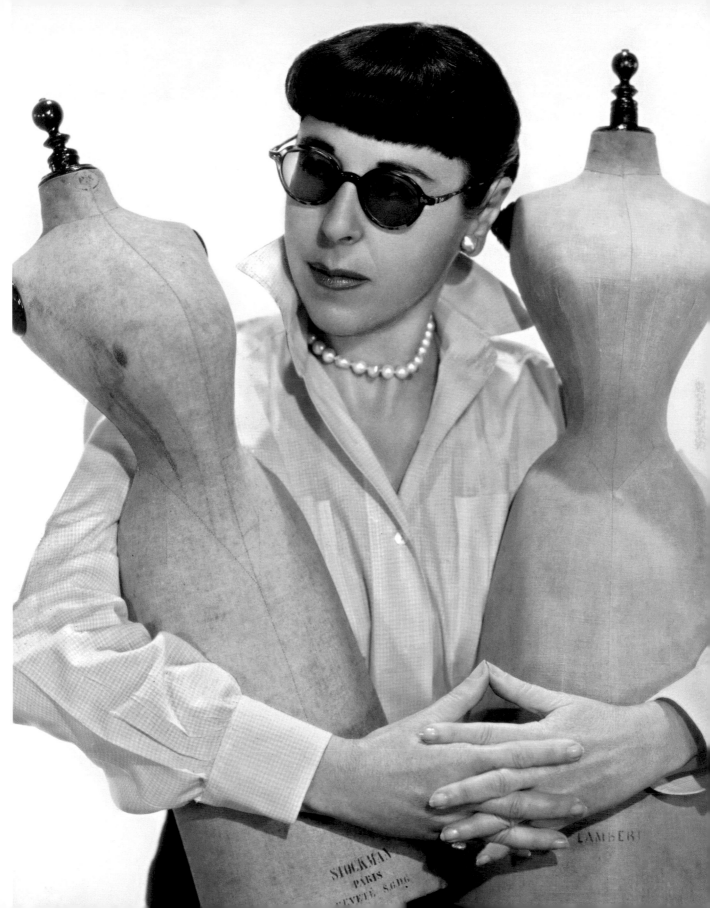

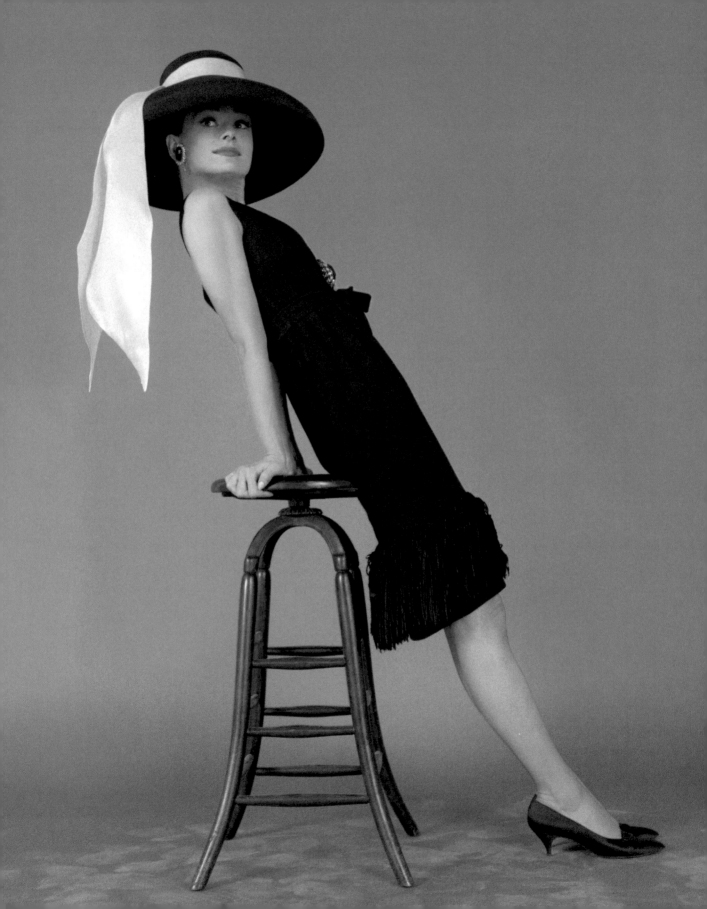

exposure and long-term appeal. Along with Helen Rose, she was only one of two female head costume designers at a major Hollywood studio.

Above all, Head's designs served the needs of the character—the principal aim of a costume designer. Costume designers were highly involved with the entire creation of a film, and read a script carefully so that the message the clothes communicated aligned with the character's persona. The costume designer believed that clothes *came from* the character. Couturiers, of course, believed pretty much the opposite: they thought of clothing as art, a manifestation of their creative vision, and very much something that could *determine* character. So it's understandable that couture's relationship with Hollywood was, at first, quite tentative.

The first couturier to feel the lure of Hollywood, however briefly, was Coco Chanel. Sam Goldwyn offered her a million dollars to work for him, and she went for it. Unfortunately, it didn't work out so well. Chanel wouldn't compromise her clothing for the needs of her character, and, unsurprisingly, collaboration didn't appeal to her, leading to disagreements with Gloria Swanson, the star of *Tonight or Never*. After a year, Chanel was back in Paris, although she did dabble in designing for French films after that.

That wasn't the curtain call for couturiers and Hollywood. When Audrey Hepburn, a star with a keen eye for fashion, requested to work with a couturier (rather than Edith Head) for her role in 1954's *Sabrina*, she jump-started the Hollywood career of Hubert de Givenchy. Both Head and Givenchy worked on the film, which features the transformation of a simple girl into a sophisticated lady—but Head was given the pre-transformation clothing, Givenchy the glamorous post-transformation wardrobe. Givenchy's gowns were stunning, and the film generated a lot of publicity for his couture house; the pairing also sparked a lifelong partnership between Hepburn and the couturier. Notably, their work on *Breakfast at Tiffany's* popularized the idea of the "little black dress," an established fashion staple today. Their collaboration also changed the way costuming worked. No longer was it purely the domain of costume departments.

By the sixties, the ready-to-wear clothing market boomed (see "Ready-to-Wear and Mass Fashion")

left — *Breakfast at Tiffany's* introduced a new fashion star: the little black dress, as worn by Audrey Hepburn—and designed, of course, by Givenchy.

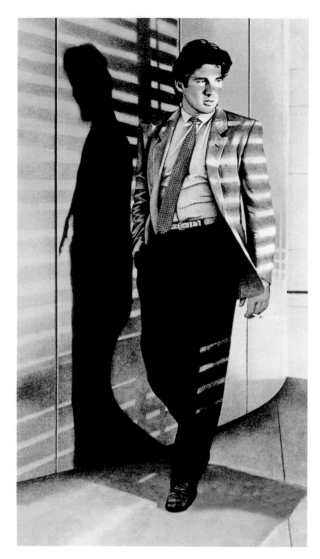

while couture was on the wane, and this was reflected in movies. It became common for ready-to-wear creations to appear in films, and, with the exception of Edith Head, head designers were a thing of the past. Instead of designing costumes in-house, most studios bought ready-to-wear. And true to the fact that very few movies since have featured traditional costume design, films set in contemporary times have rarely won Academy Awards for costume design, losing out to epics, musicals, and period pieces.

Ready-to-wear fashion had many players, but one of its biggest innovators was Giorgio Armani. He found a way to make ready-to-wear appear luxurious to the consumer—and he had some ingenious ideas about

how to market it, too. Armani slipped easily into film costuming for 1980's *American Gigolo* with Richard Gere, whose suave, slim-hipped male escort character wore ready-to-wear Armani suits like they were made for him. The film almost feels like an extended commercial for Armani clothing, but it brought the kind of widespread recognition and implicit cool that an ad never could.

But not all film fashion was off the rack. One of the great artists to work within costume design from the eighties onward has been Jean Paul Gaultier. Gaultier's couture has always skewed to the provocative and decadent (he was the one who designed Madonna's infamous cone bra), and fortunately for him, the films he's worked on (such as *The Cook, the Thief, His Wife and Her Lover, Kika, The City of Lost Children*, and *The Fifth Element*) have allowed him to put his fashion first, without making sacrifices for the sake of character. Considering his close association with film and culture, it's no surprise that Gaultier has been influenced by the medium himself; in spring 2008, he released a collection inspired

above —In *American Gigolo*, Richard Gere had hustle, at least partially due to his slick wardrobe of Armani suits.

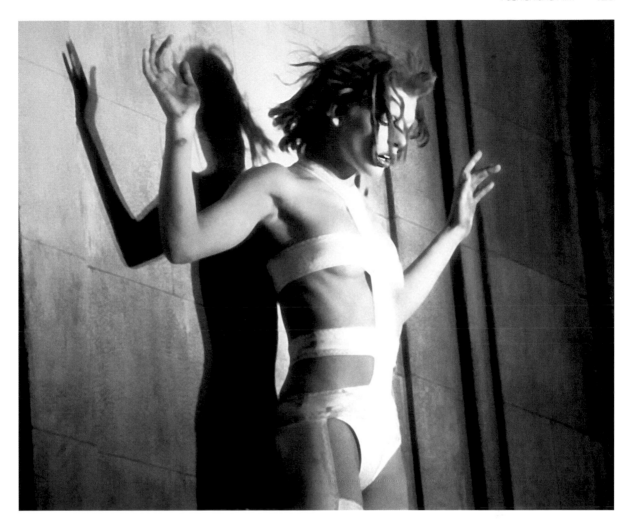

by *Pirates of the Caribbean 3*, complete with boots, buckles, and jaunty pirate hats.

These days the ties between film and fashion are so mutual and acknowledged that fashion is often a character unto itself. In swag-heavy films like *Clueless* (1995), *Sex and the City: The Movie* and its sequel (2008, 2010), *The Devil Wears Prada* (2006), and *The Bling Ring* (2013), characters openly name-check designers, and wearing major names is a heroic struggle. The two *Sex and the City* films and

The Devil Wears Prada feature costume design from Patricia Field, a stylist who has frequently been snagged as a costume designer on fashion-themed films after her success on the *Sex and the City* TV series.

And if fashion can be a character in film, it is only fair that a designer should direct. *A Single Man* of 2009 was the grand cinematic entrance of fashion designer Tom Ford, who directed, and also financed, the film (though he delegated costume design to Arianne Phillips). It received critical acclaim, and was almost unanimously declared as "beautiful," in no small part to the film's gorgeous, and very taste-ful, early-sixties-inspired clothes. Unlike *Sex and the City* or *The Devil Wears Prada*, the fashion doesn't yell, taking the quieter approach of the elegant

above — Jean Paul Gaultier's over-the-top fashion looked at home in the sci-fi spectacle of *The Fifth Element*. In this still, Milla Jovovich wears one of Gaultier's provocative designs.

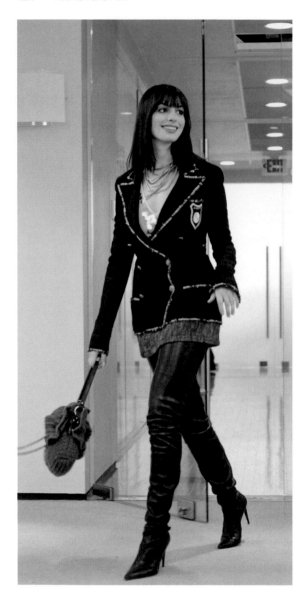

couter of the era in which it was set—no doubt subtly enhancing Tom Ford's brand image.

In the early part of the twentieth century, film's pull with popular fashion may have come as a surprise to clothing manufacturers, but not these days. For 2013's *The Great Gatsby*, the feverish adoption of flapper styles was well anticipated and planned for. Knowing the film had a spring release, many designers, including Marc Jacobs and Ralph Lauren, planned Spring 2013 lines that included nods to Roaring Twenties designs like drop-waist dresses and cloche hats. But Brooks Brothers had

even deeper ties; they not only collaborated with the film's costume designer, Catherine Martin, to create the film's wardrobe, but also released a Gatsby-themed collection to coincide with the film's release.

It's not just mega-blockbusters that feature fashion tie-ins with clothing producers; Harmony Korine's girls-gone-gangster epic *Spring Breakers* (2012) saw its costume designer collaborate on a themed collection with edgy high-fashion boutique Opening Ceremony that featured sweatpants emblazoned with glow-in-the-dark aliens and dolphins and neon leopard-print bikinis. Fashion's impulses and obsessions, whether large scale or niche, are undeniably tied to film—and in an era when films and their wardrobes are only ever a few clicks away, film has the power to influence more people than any time in its history.

above — Dropping names like they're going out of style: Anne Hathaway's character in *The Devil Wears Prada* learned to love brand-name swag.

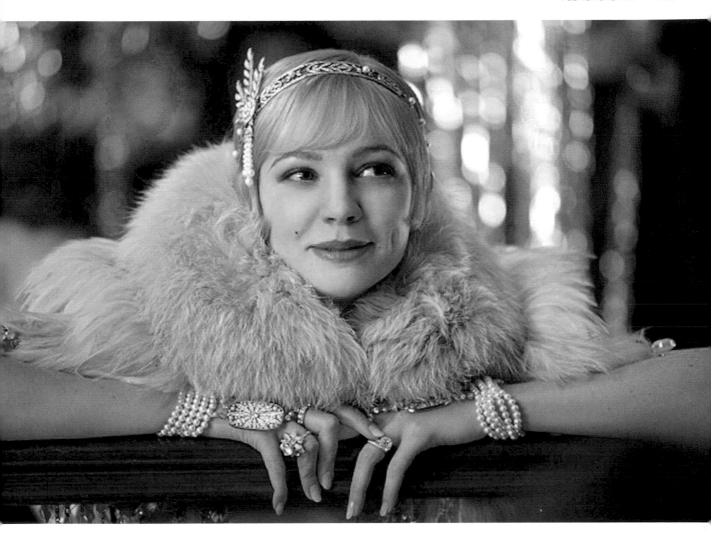

above — Why, of course you can repeat the past: the Roaring Twenties-themed fashion tie-ins for *The Great Gatsby* were planned well in advance. Shown here is Carey Mulligan in glamorous flapper style.

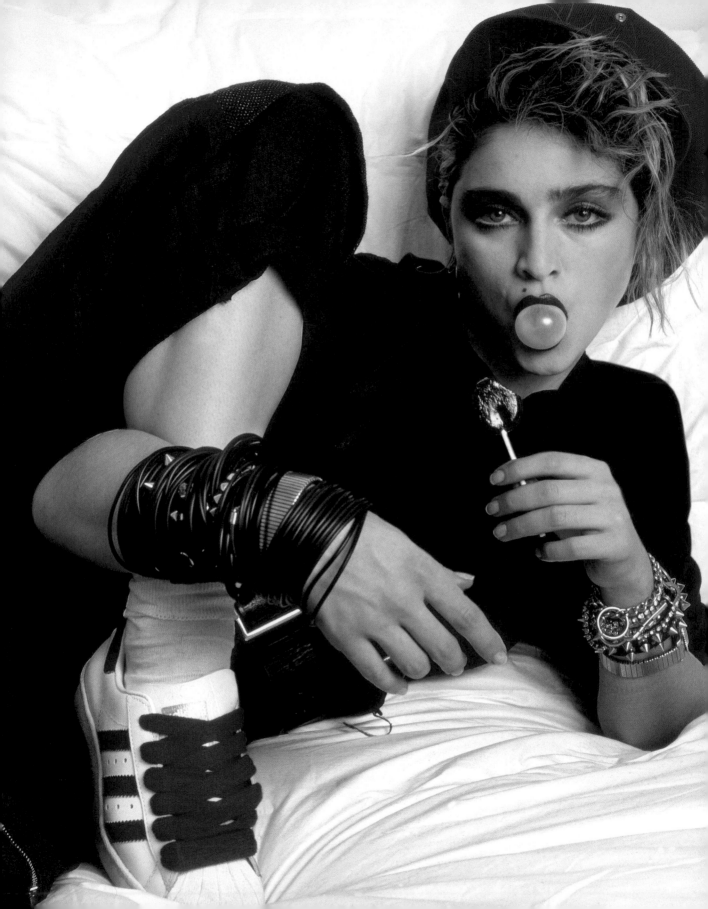

Fashion and Music

Pouting out from Saint Laurent's sultry black-and-white 2013 ad campaign is none other than Courtney Love, grunge music's still unapologetically hard-living queen. She's joined by a cadre of other musicians known for their nonconformist style: Kim Gordon, Marilyn Manson, Ariel Pink, and Daft Punk. For most modern consumers, well acquainted with the relationship between fashion and music, the aim of the ads won't be a mystery: to give the label some badass rock 'n' roll attitude. When music first began to influence fashion, it happened organically, as the rebellious lifestyles of musicians spilled over into their fashion choices. Inspiring the mimicry of fans coveting a little edge, music-influenced looks eventually become less subversive and more integrated into everyday fashion (see "Fashion Subcultures"). The first example of this came in the form of the zoot suit. A jazz-club staple of the thirties, the zoot suit was a dramatically flowing garment that emphasized a man's upper body with broad shoulders and billowing trousers that tapered at the waist. Variously attributed to places as far-flung as Chicago, New York, and Memphis, the zoot suit was mainly worn by stylish African Americans, and was popularized by musicians like Cab Calloway, Dizzy Gillespie, and Louis Armstrong in the thirties and forties. The suits soon became more streamlined, and a young Elvis Presley frequented black Memphis's preemi-nent menswear shop to buy black-and-pink drape suits that became the trademark of his early days in the fifties.

Around the same time as young men were slipping on zoot suits to cultivate a bad-boy image, the swing music of the forties provoked a fashion frenzy that lived entirely on the dance floor: bobby soxers. Bobby soxers were as known for their look—poodle skirts, ribbon-tied ponytails, and ankle socks—as for their ardent love of Frank Sinatra. Sinatra was so adored by the bobby soxers that he required a police guard in public to hold back the poodle-skirted teenagers; young men, hoping to sponge off his popularity, copied his polka-dotted tie.

Over-the-top female fans were also a signature of one of the sixties most sartorially significant groups: the Beatles. The Beatle style was a variation on the fashion-conscious mod look common in Britain at the time. The band became known for their "Beatle

left — Layered bangles, heavy eyeliner, and obvious 'tude: in the early 1980s, every teen mallrat wanted to look like Madonna.

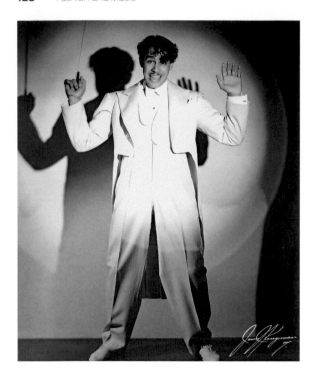

cut" hairstyle (originally the work of one of the band members' girlfriends), as well as their collarless suits, dreamed up by their manager Brian Epstein. Designed by Ted Lapidus, the suits became de rigueur for bands hoping to profit off the popularity of Beatlemania.

Often cast as the yin to the Beatles' yang, the Rolling Stones started off dressing somewhat like the Fab Four, but soon ditched the neat suits for more overtly bohemian attire—scarves, eyeliner, and floppy velvet hats, a style which became the visual definition of a glamorous, drug-fueled rock 'n' roll lifestyle. Their look was the brilliant creation of Keith Richards's girlfriend, Anita Pallenberg, who became a fashion icon for her creative outfitting of the band and herself.

By the late sixties, hippie culture was shaping youth fashion in a major way, and many of its idols were musicians; one of the most influential was Janis Joplin. Joplin epitomized the exotic thrift-store ethos of the hippie look: she wore silks, leathers, and velvets, did some of her own sewing, layered everything with beads and jewelry, and perched ostrich feathers in her hair. This carefree, bohemian look

was seen everywhere during the hippie era, and in particularly high concentrations at music festivals like Woodstock.

The folksy hippie scene saw its inevitable fashion backlash in the hard-edged, antiauthoritarian punk movement. Punk's genesis was in New York, but the place where it really seized fashion was London, due to the efforts of the business-minded artistic provocateur Malcolm McLaren. Beginning in 1971, McLaren operated a clothing store (which frequently changed its name) on Kings Road with his then girlfriend Vivienne Westwood. After a sojourn in New York managing the New York Dolls, McLaren and Westwood began to supply clothing to the band, renaming their store SEX in 1974. SEX sold clothing, designed by Westwood, that appealed to London's young punks—styles inspired by fetish and bondage wear using rubber, lacing, and dog collars, mostly in black.

McLaren's most innovative and genre-defining move, however, was to create a band called the Sex Pistols, brazenly named after his shop. He recruited his front man from the shop's clientele: John Lydon, who McLaren remade as Johnny Rotten. McLaren

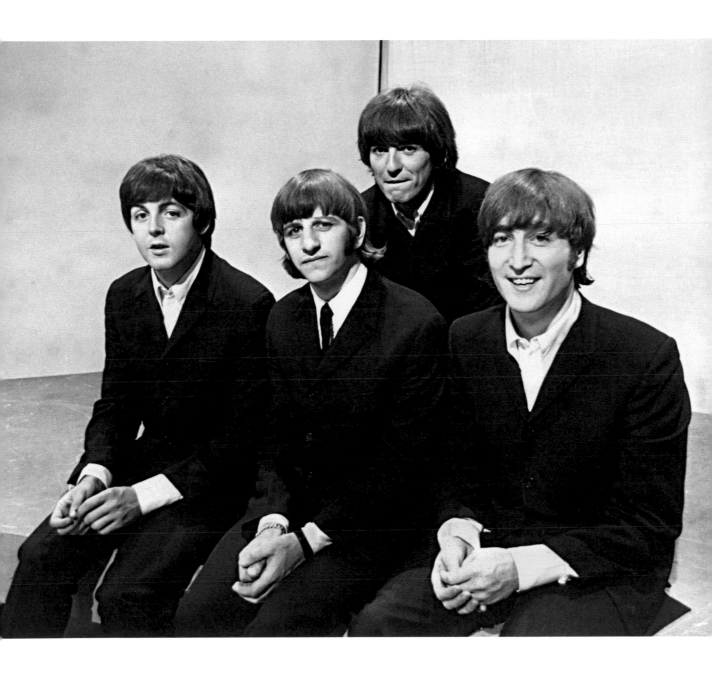

left — He had flow, and so did his clothes: Jazz bandleader Cab
Calloway wore his zoot suit with obvious panache.

above — Fab, for sure: the four Beatles show off their soon-
to-be iconic suits and haircuts at the BBC in 1966.

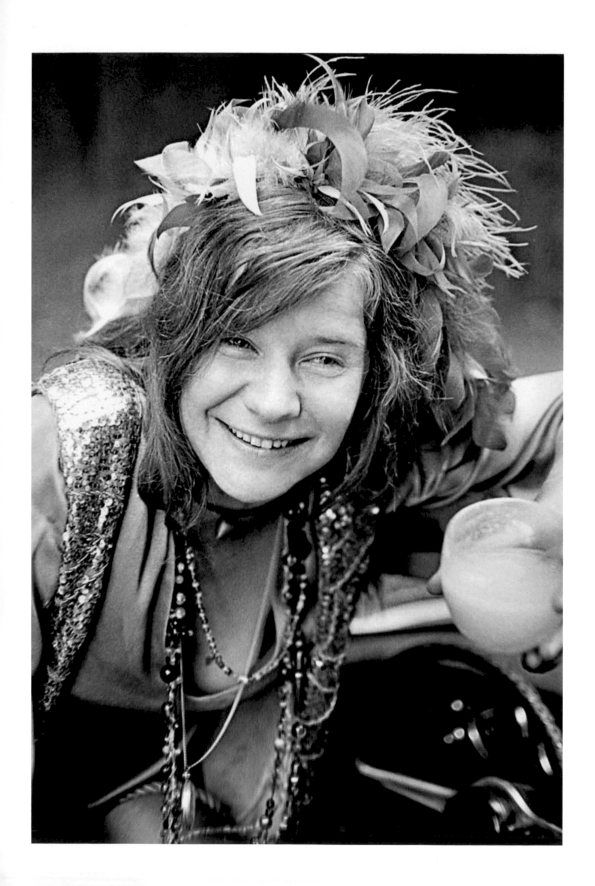

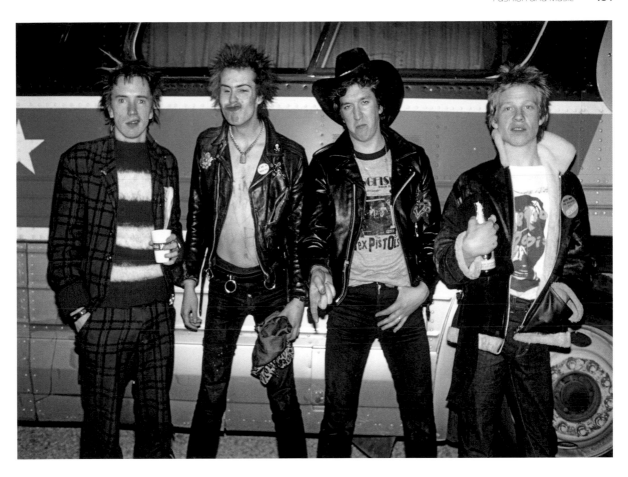

dressed the entire band in clothing from SEX, thus defining the aesthetic and commercializing it in one fell swoop. Vivienne Westwood, meanwhile, became the person to legitimize punk as a high-fashion form, expanding her designs into runway fashion with a radical aesthetic that remains popular today. At around the same time as McLaren and Westwood were defining the punk look, glam rock was introducing its glitter-strewn androgyny into the

left — With her unforgettable voice and carefree, bohemian style, Janis Joplin was the queen of hippie fashion.

above — Boasting punk posturing and a wardrobe to match, the Sex Pistols (photographed here in 1978) were the genius creation of Malcolm McLaren.

public imagination. The king of glam rock was David Bowie, who delivered his high-minded, conceptual vision using an alter ego named Ziggy Stardust. Face paint, metallic pants, glitter, and platform boots were all within Ziggy's realm, with many of his looks pulled right from the ready-to-wear collection of designer Kansai Yamamoto. Later in the seventies, glam's showy looks paved the way for the peacocky styles of disco, best captured by John Travolta's sidewalk strut to the Bee Gees' hit "Stayin' Alive" in the disco-centric film *Saturday Night Fever*. Disco was responsible for bringing dance-floor fashions like flared pants, synthetic fabrics, and jumpsuits onto the streets.

By the eighties, fashion got a little darker with the advent of goth. Goth music emerged from post-punk in the eighties as a brooding musical form led by bands like Bauhaus and Siouxsie and the

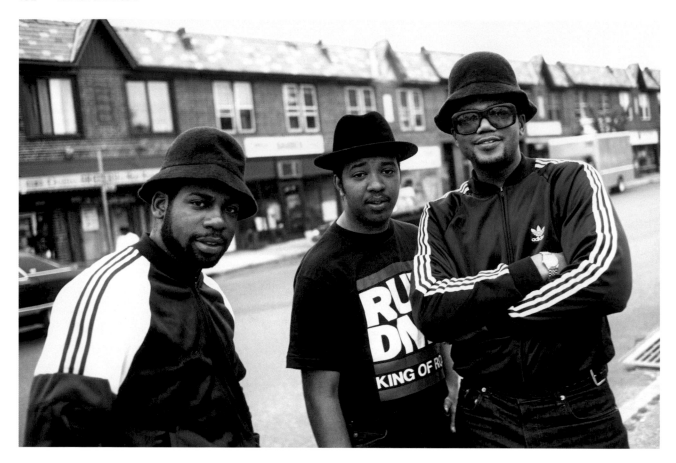

Banshees, and later on The Cure. Goth bands wore dark colors, dramatic, backcombed black hair, and heavy makeup. With its moodily theatrical aesthetic and introspective lyrics, an entire subculture of self-declared outcasts and misfits formed around goth, donning fashions inspired by the Elizabethan and Victorian eras, as well as anything considered dark or occult. To this day, goth-inspired fashion is a recurring motif in haute couture; both Alexander McQueen (prior to his death) and Jean Paul Gaultier have been slapped with the label of "haute goth" for their dark, historically inspired designs.

A rising force in eighties fashion was hip-hop, which bubbled up from the underground to achieve widespread popularity. The look's forerunners were Run-DMC, who moved hip-hop's aesthetics away from the flashy, disco style worn by acts like Grandmaster Flash toward a more street-influenced look involving sportswear, gold chains, fedoras, and Adidas shoes (see "Sports and Fashion"). Run-DMC immortalized their shoe fixation with the song "My Adidas," and active sportswear dominated hip-hop fashion thereafter. Capitalizing on hip-hop's nascent sway over fashion was Def Jam magnate Russell Simmons, who founded one of the first celebrity-fronted fashion labels, Phat Farm, in 1992 (see "Celebrity Fashion"). Phat Farm promoted a preppier version of hip-hop fashion, appropriating the Ivy League aesthetic and making it a little more street.

above — They loved their Adidas, but Run-DMC's influence on fashion went far beyond shoes.

right — Nirvana channeled teenage angst into fashion, bringing popularity to the layered grunge style. The band is shown here in Belfast in 1992.

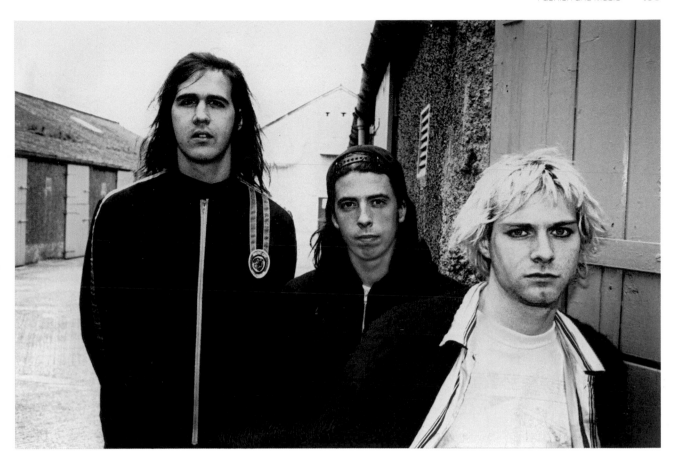

When it comes to women's fashion in the eighties, the influence of Madonna is undeniable. Her early look—lace tops, rubber bracelets, crucifix jewelry, hairsprayed hair, and fishnet stockings—was a favorite of teen mallrats trying to cultivate a little attitude. The look was conceived by Madonna's stylist at the time, Maripol, a jewelry designer. Madonna's chameleonic, influential style particularly appealed to one designer, Jean Paul Gaultier, who saw her as an ideal collaborator. During her *Blonde Ambition* tour of the nineties, Gaultier began designing for her, cementing infamy for both of them by dressing her in his soon-to-be-iconic cone bra.

In the nineties, a rather aesthetically unpretentious subculture changed the course of fashion—grunge. Springing up in the gray, chilly climate of the Pacific Northwest, grunge was a fuzzy, distorted style of rock music epitomized by bands like Nirvana, Pearl Jam, Soundgarden, and Hole. The look of grunge

bands was more practical than statement-making. It featured layered, outdoorsy clothing that suited the rainy, temperate climate: stonewashed jeans, plaid work shirts (sometimes worn tied around the waist), band T-shirts, and Doc Martens. The more feminine "kinderwhore" look, a staple of nineties-era female wardrobes, was popularized by Courtney Love of Hole and Kat Bjelland of Babes in Toyland, juxtaposing innocence with overt sexuality by pairing short, floral babydoll dresses with boots and heavy makeup. Easily and cheaply emulated, the grunge aesthetic achieved mass mainstream popularity, and was an inspiration for fashion designers such as Marc Jacobs, who brought its ethos to high-end fashion.

In the tradition of fashion provocateurs like David Bowie and Madonna, today Lady Gaga makes intentionally shocking fashion choices to build her stage persona. Two particularly provocative fashion

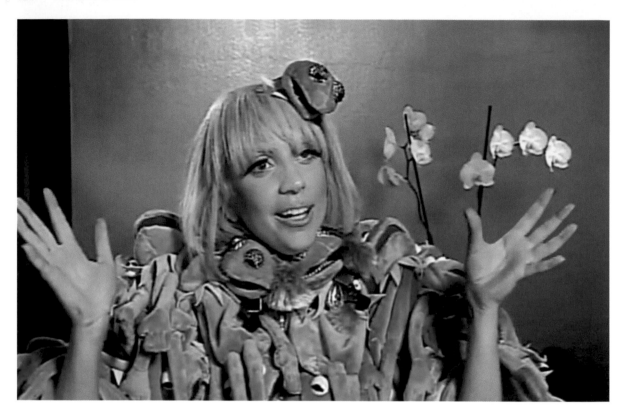

examples from Gaga's aesthetic oeuvre include her Kermit the Frog coat, designed by Jean-Charles de Castelbajac, which she wore on German TV in 2009, and the "meat dress" designed by the Haus of Gaga, which she wore to great furor at the 2010 MTV Video Music Awards. Gaga's theatrical and over-the-top looks are all part of her effort to create a character, but her popular appeal and wild choices have turned her into an inspiration for fashion designers: looks that appear to be derived from her costumes have shown up on the runways of designers as disparate as Derek Lam, Prada, Alexander Wang, and Rodarte.

In the present day, fashion's relationship with music is well established and often highly manipulated—far from music's early, natural influence on fashion. Musicians expand their brands by fronting fashion lines (Diddy's Sean John, Beyonce's House of Deréon, and Gwen Stefani's L.A.M.B. are all examples), designers carefully choose runway soundtracks to give their collection the right mood, and major labels place musicians in their ads to appear appealingly bohemian, rather than corporate. But as a medium that thrives on creativity and nonconformity, music still offers plenty of uncorrupted fashion inspiration to fans. It's a personal choice whether they copy the look with the mediation of a major fashion label, or do it the really rock 'n' roll way—independently.

above — Muppets were harmed in the making of this coat: Lady Gaga shows off her Kermit coat (designed by Jean-Charles de Castelbajac) on German TV.

right — Confrontationally sexy, Courtney Love rocks the "kinderwhore" look in 1993.

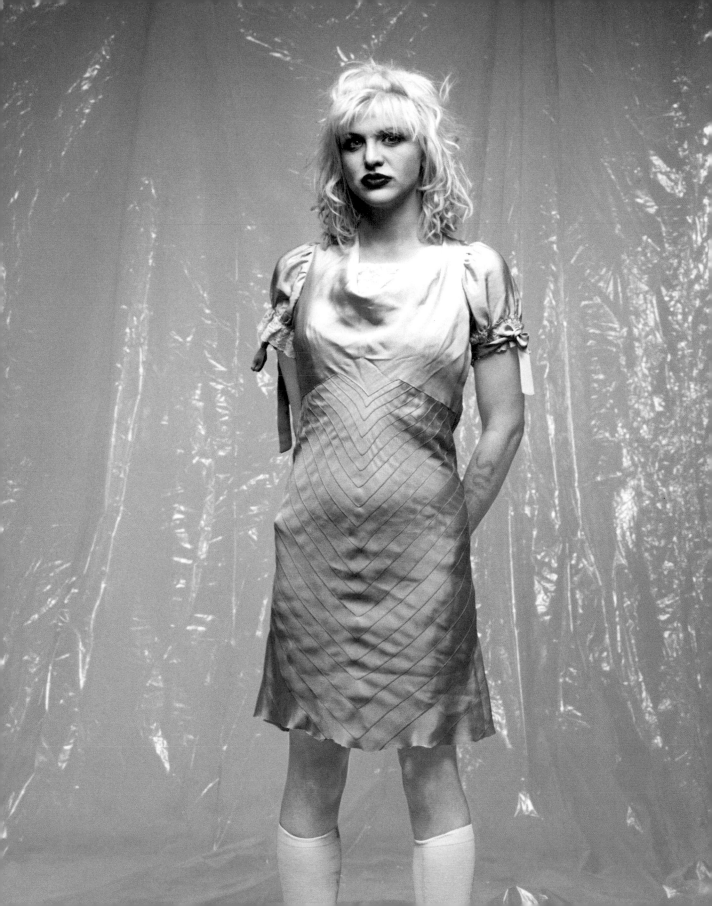

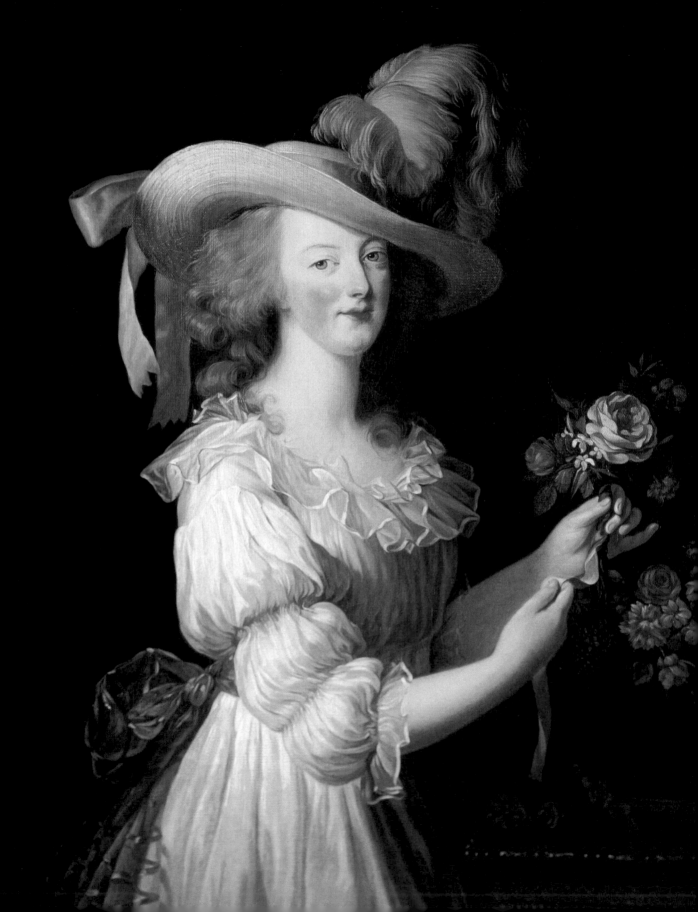

Celebrity Fashion

Hoisting canapés, quaffing cocktails, and hovering over Twitter on smartphones: this is the average person's itinerary at an Oscar party. On the day of the Academy Awards, the celebration starts an hour or so before the actual awards ceremony begins so that guests can variously swoon or groan over the red-carpet fashions. Stars vamp and namedrop "who" they're wearing: Alexander McQueen, Valentino, Gucci, Dior. It's an event that inspires more gossip, press, and accolades than even the most dramatic couture presentations in Paris, and it's all due to the power of celebrity.

In a way, fashion has always been linked to celebrity; historically, the rich and powerful were the ones with the funds and influence to shape trends. Marie Antoinette was known across Europe for her elaborate, often controversial fashions, and women specifically aspired to her look, purchasing clothing from her purveyors and getting stylists to copy her hairstyles (see "Royal Fashion"). But Marie Antoinette was different from modern celebrities: she was indisputably an important person (not a prerequisite for fame now), yet the reach of her fame wasn't as broad as that of celebrities today. Modern celebrities emerged alongside print and movies, which allowed for the mass production (and mass consumption) of culture. Often, the subjects of public admiration were monarchs, society ladies, and actresses: the flashiest jobs of the time. Print and film culture coincided, roughly, with the invention of couture (see "Couture"), and one of the first major celebrities to be dressed by the couturiers was the reigning queen of the stage, actress Sarah Bernhardt. In the late nineteenth century, the house of Jacques Doucet handled much of her costuming (driving his business with the exposure this provided), and eventually she was passed along to Doucet's skilled assistant, the soon to be notorious Paul Poiret. Poiret designed for her successfully until she caught him making fun of her for wearing slacks in her role as Napoleon's son in *L'Aiglon* in 1898, at which point he was summarily fired.

Beginning in the 1920s, the golden age of Hollywood and its star system brought more power and exposure to celebrities. Film stars were groomed by the studios and celebrated as icons, often with a fashionable image (see "Fashion and Film"). With

left — It's not easy being queen: Marie Antoinette's fashions helped her achieve celebrity—and also ensured her downfall. This painting by Louise Élisabeth Vigée Le Brun depicts her in 1783.

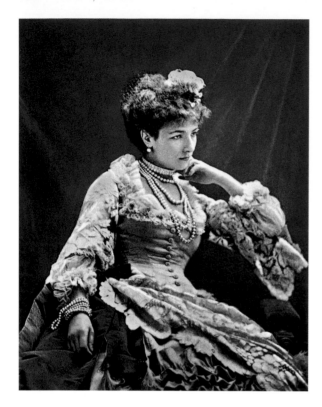

left — During her reign of the stage, actress Sarah Bernhardt (shown here in 1860) was declared "the most famous actress the world has ever known." Her palpable celebrity brought many customers to the House of Doucet, who designed much of her clothing.

that power came the ability to influence trends. One prime example of this star power at work came via Marlene Dietrich, a glamorous cabaret performer who transitioned to the silver screen in the thirties. Dietrich was vampy, but her style was often masculine. She favored square shoulders, suits, and tuxedos, and, along with Katharine Hepburn, helped to inspire women to put on trousers.

A bigger fashion sensation was lithe, pert-nosed brunette Audrey Hepburn. Quirky and upbeat, Hepburn had a natural sense of style, and suggested, for her role in the 1954 film *Sabrina*, that rather than be dressed by Hollywood's top stylist, Edith Head, she wear real Parisian couture. Her initial appointment was with Balenciaga, but he passed her on to Givenchy, a fortunate pairing that sparked one of fashion's longest and most notable collaborations, predating designer/muse relationships like that of Hermès and Jane Birkin and Marc Jacobs and Sofia Coppola.

It's impossible to talk about celebrity fashion without at least touching on Marilyn Monroe. Monroe was a creation of Norma Jeane Mortenson:

a character she acted out for the duration of her short life in the public eye in the fifties and sixties. Marilyn Monroe was a blonde bombshell whose every fashion choice was made to accentuate her sex appeal. Her low-cut dresses (which she was often sewn into), her decision to wear dresses without underwear (to avoid lines), her red lips, and her kittenish demeanor were all tools she deployed to build a character. It's a strategy that was echoed a few decades later, by both Madonna (in the eighties) and Lady Gaga (in the aughts).

Things changed after Hollywood's golden age. In the seventies and eighties, culture became much more commodified, and celebrities grew ever more

right — Marlene Dietrich's on-screen fame helped squeeze women into trousers. She's photographed here in 1932.

next pages — Givenchy's celebrity muse Audrey Hepburn (shown here in a promotional shot for *Sabrina*) popularized the French couturier among the masses.

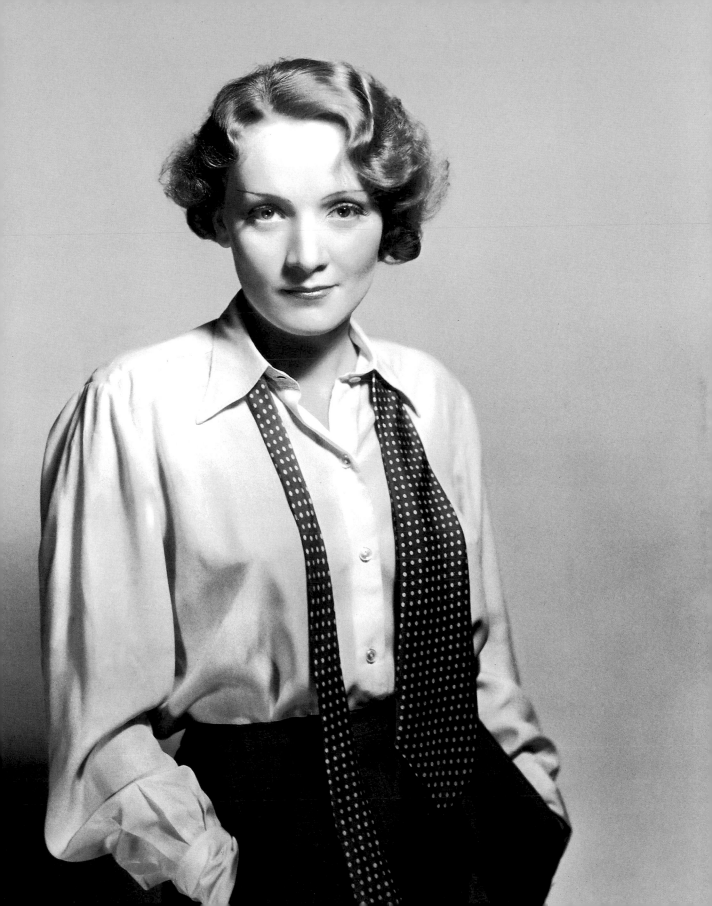

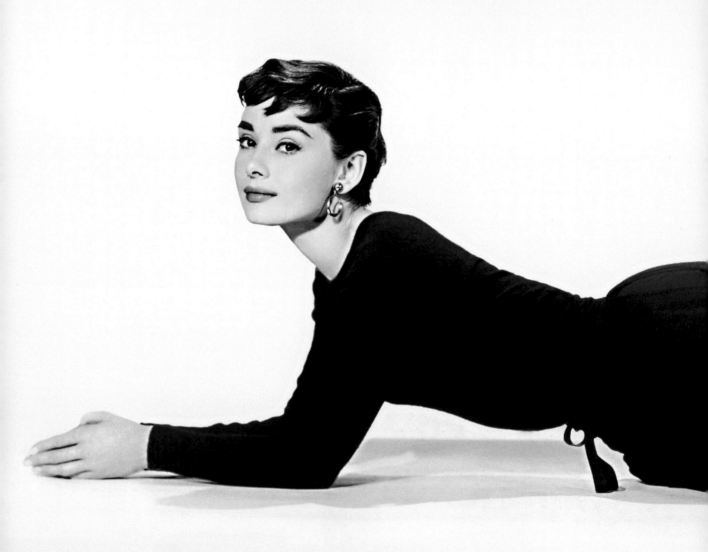

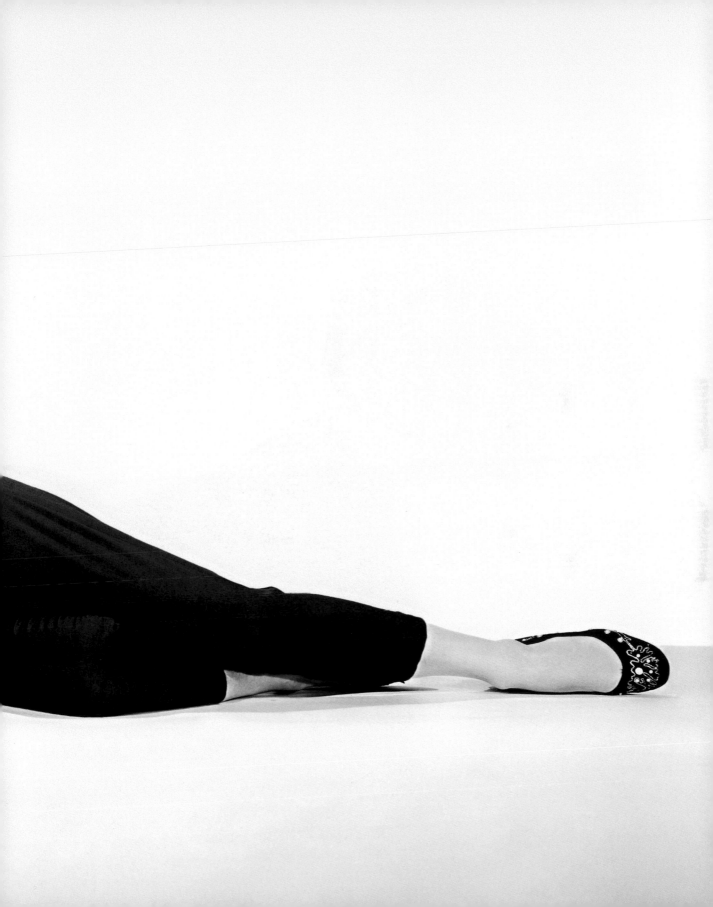

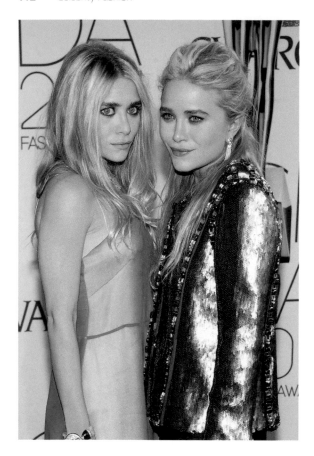

powerful. In the process, they transitioned into marketing tools: brands in and of themselves. And so it was only natural that celebrities would begin to launch their own clothing lines. One early example was Gloria Vanderbilt, the glamorous American heiress/actress. In the seventies, after experimenting with licensing her name to a line of scarves, she began to design blue jeans: a tight-fitting jean with her name on the back pocket. The line expanded to include dresses, and she also lent her name to perfumes, all successful ventures.

In the late nineties and early aughts, there was an explosion of celebrity-fronted fashion brands. Phat Farm, Def Jam record magnate Russell Simmons's sportswear line, has been a successful example since 1992; Jay-Z followed with his brand, Rocawear, in 1999. When it comes to higher-end fashion, Mary-Kate and Ashley Olsen have had great success with their lines The Row and Elizabeth and James; Nicole Richie has been similarly successful with Winter

Kate and House of Harlow 1960. These days, it's so common for celebrities to own fashion labels (whether mass-market or higher end) that it's practically more of a surprise when they aren't designing fashion. It's barely worth a raised eyebrow that reality stars the Kardashians have their own line at Sears (the Kardashian Kollection). Of course, the fashion world takes the Olsens and Richie more seriously; they're genuinely interested in fashion culture and design, which isn't a given for celebrity designers. Perhaps the most important development in celebrity fashion in the twenty-first century has been the rise of the stylist. Once, celebrities became fashion icons because they had a legitimate sense of style,

above — They got it, dude: lifelong stars Mary-Kate and Ashley Olsen (shown here in 2011) design two of the most legitimate celeb-fronted lines, The Row and Elizabeth and James.

as in the case of Audrey Hepburn. These days, most celebrities don't dress themselves, handing that duty off to stylists—who in turn have cozy relationships with designers and brands that they need to represent on their clients. Style, these days, isn't always a personal choice.

One of the most famous celebrity stylists is Rachel Zoe, whose clients (including Nicole Richie, Keira Knightley, and Lindsay Lohan) became so well known for wearing Zoe's "boho-chic" look, with flowing curls, loose clothing, enormous sunglasses, and a gaunt frame, that they were nicknamed the "Zoe-bots" in the mid-aughts. Since then, Zoe has become a fashion celebrity in her own right, with a TV show on Bravo and her own celebrity fashion label, Luxe Rachel Zoe, sold on the QVC channel. Another stylist phenomenon is Nicola Formichetti, whose fame is tethered to that of Lady Gaga. Gaga, whose real name is Stefani Germanotta, uses fashion to shape her edgy stage persona (her legions of followers mimic her wild looks, calling themselves "Little Monsters"). Her choices are risky and

provocative; the "meat dress" (made from raw flank steak) that she wore to the 2010 MTV Video Music Awards is still notorious—a product of the Haus of Gaga, the creative team fronted by Formichetti that designs many of Gaga's looks and props. Gaga met Formichetti (then a magazine stylist) in 2009 on a fashion shoot for *V*. Ever since, her appearance has been a collaboration between the two. Formichetti's exposure via Gaga's celebrity has cemented his role in the fashion world; he recently took a gig as the

above — I, Zoe-bot: celebrity stylist Rachel Zoe has found fame styling young stars in her likeness.

creative director for Thierry Mugler, before leaving to become the artistic director at Diesel in 2013. More so than ever, these days celebrity fashion is openly used as a marketing tool. A good example is the show *Gossip Girl*, which aimed to mimic the fashion-driven success of *Sex and the City* (which turned its Manolo Blahnik-loving heroine Carrie Bradshaw's actress, Sarah Jessica Parker, into a much-loved fashion celebrity in the late nineties). But from its debut in 2007, *Gossip Girl* was blatantly commercial. The show explicitly sought to become a marketing vehicle for fashion, charging large fees for brands to appear on the show and featuring shopping advice on its website. And it succeeded: the show became one of the biggest fashion influences on young women from 2008 through 2013, and transformed its stars, Leighton Meester and Blake Lively, into fashion celebrities. Both regularly turn up as celebrity guests at fashion weeks—in fact, Lively appeared in the front row, right beside Anna Wintour, at Christian Dior's Paris Fashion Week show in 2010.

At all the major fashion weeks these days, the front rows are stacked with celebrities—not because the celebrities need a particularly good view of the runways (the fashion journalists arguably deserve that), but so that the photographers can capture these stars alongside the fashion, amping up publicity. Celebs are photographed outside venues, too, in their street clothing, often proving as much an attraction as the actual catwalk designs. It's the flipside of the red carpet, where the celebrities themselves are often upstaged by their dresses. Is it more important that Jennifer Lawrence won Best Actress at the 2012 Academy Awards, or that she wore a dramatic, cascading Dior gown? Would Marc Jacobs's 2013 fall fashion presentation at New York Fashion Week have been as compelling if Miley Cyrus and Christina Ricci weren't there? It's a question that's almost impossible to answer—and separating fashion from celebrity, and the authentic from the manufactured, will be a fashionista's dilemma for the foreseeable future.

right — Blake Lively spurred gossip when the celebrity landed front row at Paris Fashion Week in 2011, right next to Anna Wintour.

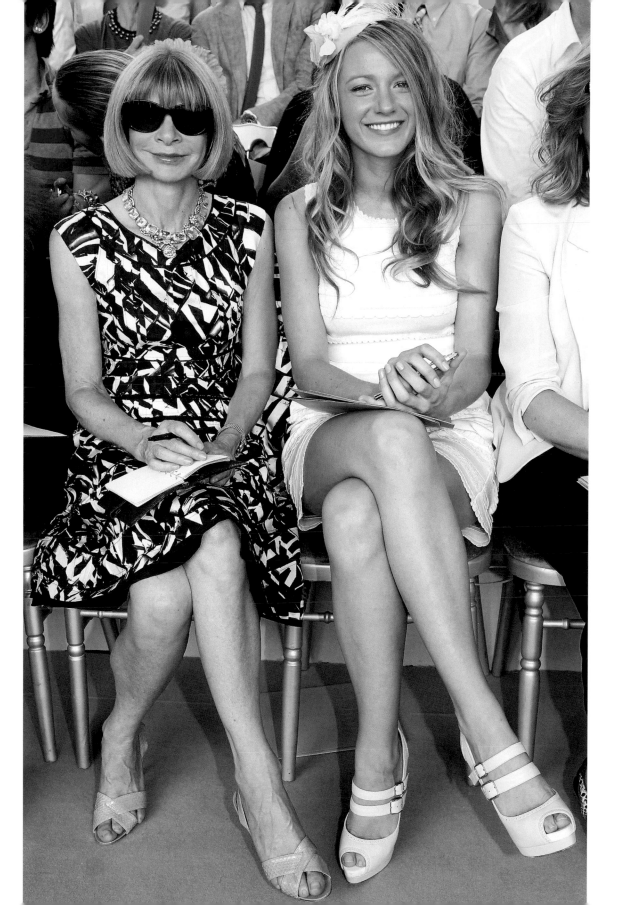

Gay and Lesbian Fashion

Makeovers are a favorite reality television theme, and one of the most well-known shows of this subgenre debuted in 2003: *Queer Eye for the Straight Guy*. The show centered around a panel of five gay men (the "Fab Five") who would overhaul the look of some regrettably unstylish straight fellow. It was instantly popular, and the five panelists became gay icons. Of course, the show depended on one key assumption: that gay men have dramatically better fashion sense than straight men. Whether that's true is debatable. But the influence of LGBT people on fashion is not. Possibly more than any other group in society, they have remained acutely aware of how their clothing affects others' perception of them. Throughout most of modern history, after all, gays and lesbians were persecuted for their lifestyles, and had to live underground— fashion was the only way they could silently communicate their orientation.

One of the earliest ways that gays and lesbians identified themselves via style was by cross-dressing. In the eighteenth century, "molly houses" (named for "mollies," slang for gay men) began to appear in London, operating like proto-gay bars where men frequently wore women's clothes. Women cross-dressed as well, though not always to attract women: often it was to escape restrictive gender norms of the time. The bisexual French writer George Sand, prolific and successful in the nineteenth century, is an example of this.

Gay subcultures emerged in various big cities by the nineteenth century, at which time fashion was becoming an established way to define one's character: the fastidious dandies of the eighteenth century (see "Menswear") had certainly set a precedent for that. It was around this time, as well, that researchers began to regard homosexuality more seriously. The nascent gay subculture was starting to mature, and one of the early events that shaped its sartorial leanings were the trials of the famous author Oscar Wilde. Wilde was an aesthete, believing that art was about celebrating the beautiful; he was also gay, and adopted a green carnation to signal his orientation. He is sometimes described as a dandy, for his interest in clothing and appearance, but Wilde's dress is equally indebted to the Aesthetic movement: clean lines, beautiful fabric, long hair, and luxurious silk

right — Smoke and mirrors: before Yves Saint Laurent's revolutionary "Le Smoking," a woman in a suit was usually considered to be cross-dressing. Here, a model poses in pinstriped YSL in 1967.

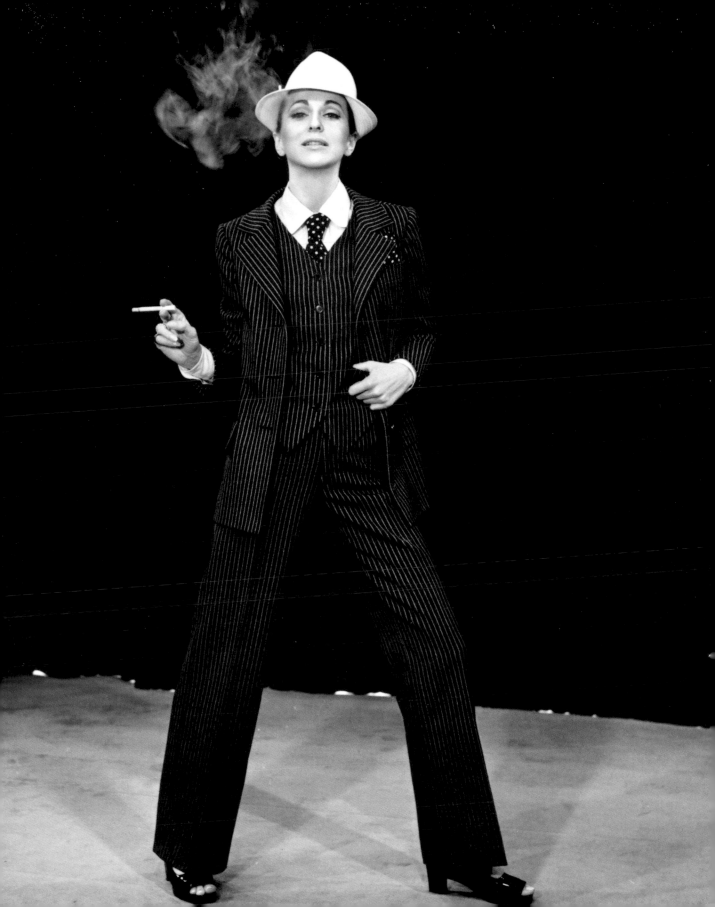

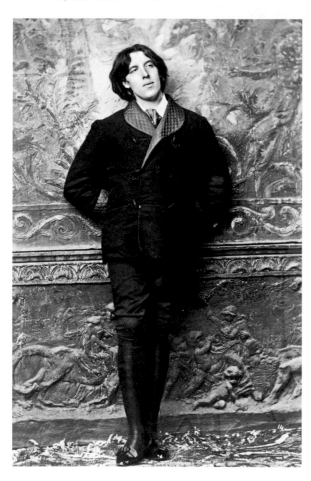

introduced the English-speaking world to Colette, exemplified the style with its neat menswear tailoring and short hairstyles. By the thirties, bisexual film stars Marlene Dietrich (whom the studios proclaimed as "The woman even women can adore") and Greta Garbo were strutting their stuff in tuxedos, which both shocked and titillated the public (see "Fashion and Film"). This look didn't fully reach the mainstream until 1966, when the woman-in-tuxedo was recognized in fashion with Yves Saint Laurent's "Le Smoking" suit.

Of course, cross-dressing was a very obvious way of declaring sexual preference, and for the better part of the twentieth century it certainly wasn't safe for everyday attire. Like Wilde's carnation, homosexual signifiers were often subtle flourishes that wouldn't be noticed by oblivious straight people. Red neckties were one symbol used up until World War II; similarly, suede shoes were a gay wardrobe staple in the thirties, but by the fifties they had lost their homosexual undertones (though still considered edgy, as

stockings. Over three highly public trials in 1895, Wilde was tried for charges of gross indecency, with the newspapers printing then-scandalous details of his entanglements with younger men. The trials cemented in the public imagination the image of gay men as fashion-conscious aesthetes.

By the twentieth century, masquerade balls had become a refuge for gays and lesbians looking for a place to let down their guard. In the twenties, the Hamilton Lodge Ball in Harlem was one of the best known; by the eighties, ball culture had evolved, and so-called houses held balls where performers would compete against each to prove the "realness" of their drag—a scene immortalized in the 1990 documentary film *Paris Is Burning*.

In between the two world wars, an era known for the rise of flappers and a more androgynous style for females (see "Fashion Subcultures"), lesbian attire flourished. Una Troubridge, a translator who

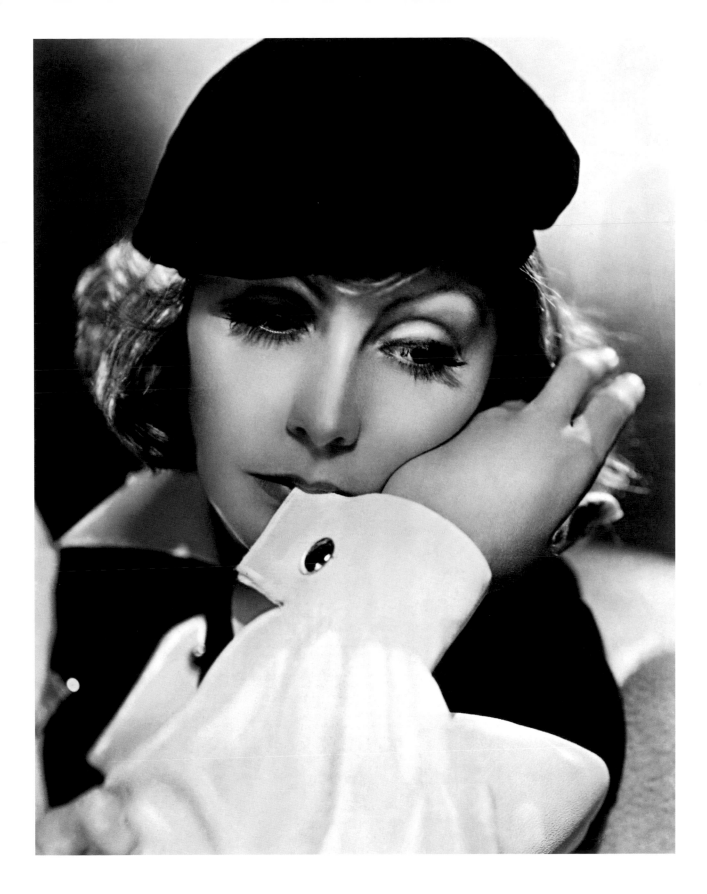

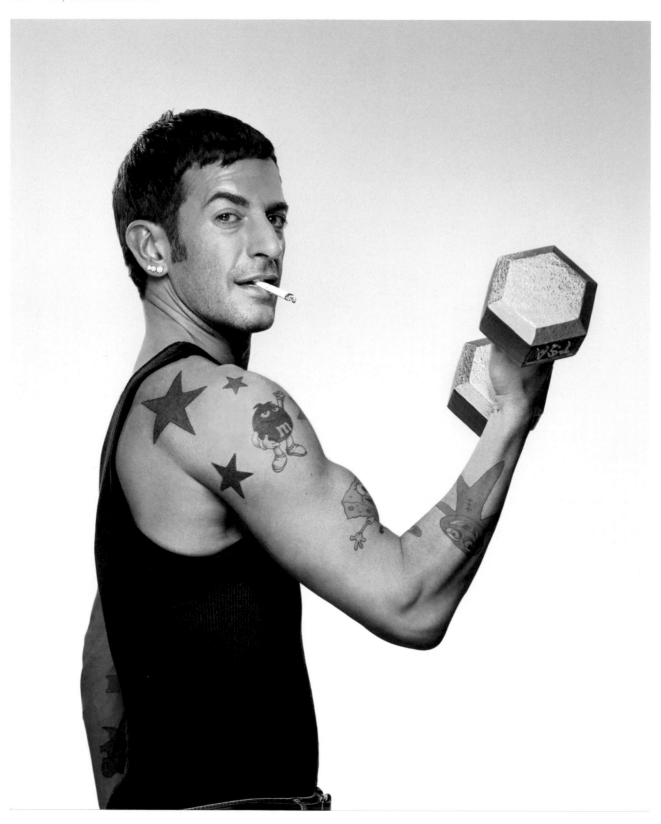

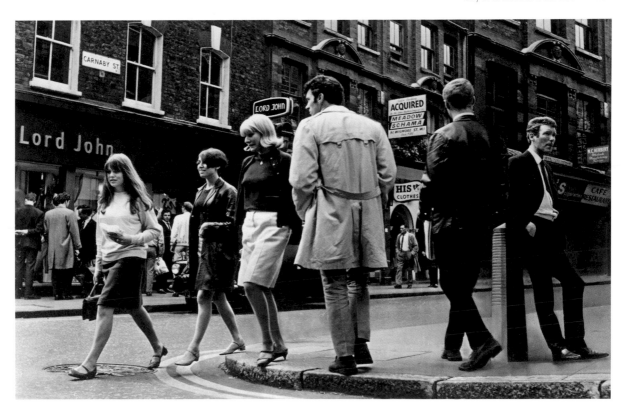

evidenced by Carl Perkins's lyrics for "Blue Suede Shoes"). Even later in the twentieth century, when homosexuality was more accepted, subtle signifiers still existed: in the S&M leather community, wearing keys on one or the other side of the belt chain indicated whether someone was submissive or dominant, while a handkerchief in a certain color in either the left or back pocket indicated a wide range of peccadilloes.

The mid-twentieth century, with its youth cultural revolution (see "Fashion Subcultures"), provided the easiest opportunity for gay fashion to influence

straight fashion, as people searched for new and different ways to subvert their wardrobes. Some major inspiration came from a Soho menswear shop called Vince. Vince's owner, Bill Green, had formerly specialized in physique photography, which captured the male physique in athletic poses—often a sly way of evading laws banning pornographic images of men. During his travels Green had been inspired by continental fashions, and for Vince he designed close-fitting, colorful designs in velvet and silk that sold to an artsy crowd well populated with gay clientele. One of Green's shop assistants opened his own store, His Clothes, on Carnaby Street, modeled after Vince. His Clothes was the store that kicked off the boom of shops on Carnaby Street, ultimately feeding the mod fashion phenomenon, and later, hippie fashions.

By the seventies, as straight style more closely resembled what had formerly been gay fashion, gay men began to wear more stereotypically masculine attire: and so the "clone" was born. These looks, too, found their way into popular fashions: handlebar

above — Carnaby Street, it turns out, may need to write a thank-you card to gay culture. The fashionable shopping street is shown here at the height of Swinging London in 1965.

left — Fashion heavyweight Marc Jacobs (photographed here by Martin Schoeller) is just one of many influential gay designers.

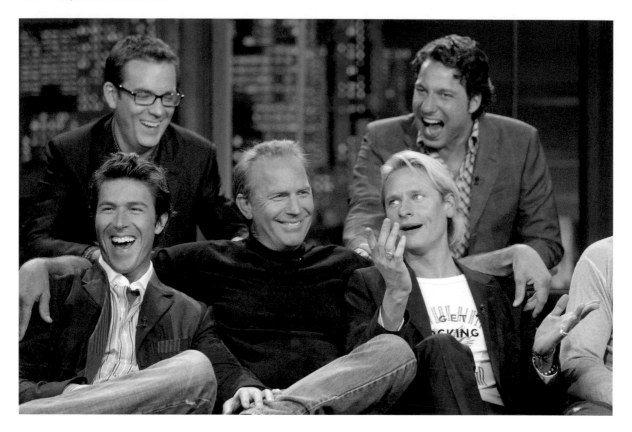

moustaches and Levi's 501s are as much a symbol of the seventies as they are of masculinity. Around the same time, the women's rights movement was taking off (see "Feminism and Fashion"), accompanied by Saint Laurent's "Le Smoking" tuxedo, and what had once been a stereotypically lesbian look was the stuff of mainstream fashion magazines.

The latter half of the twentieth century marked the beginning of the gay rights movement. Notably, fashion designer Rudi Gernreich helped found the Mattachine Society, one of America's first homosexual organizations, in 1950. Gernreich later became known for his unisex fashions, as well as his infamous monokini, while the Mattachine Society declined after the Stonewall Riots of 1969 and the emergence of more militant rights organizations such as the Gay Liberation Front.

Post-Stonewall, gays and lesbians were more visible in society—and at the same time, many of the fashions that had originally defined them became more mainstream. In particular, androgyny came to the fore in fashion, and boyish girls like Twiggy and girlish boys like David Bowie or Mick Jagger were leading trends.

In the eighties, crisis hit the gay community with the devastation of AIDS. There was a backlash in gay fashion, with the S&M influenced "leatherman" style becoming passé. Beyond gay-specific fashions, AIDS struck the fashion industry right to its core: its losses included Perry Ellis, who succumbed to AIDS in 1986, and Halston, who passed away in 1990, as well as a raft of young talent. That year, newspaper reports detailed the extent of fashion's vulnerability to AIDS: a large percentage of the industry's talent was gay, making the disease a huge concern. And while, fortunately, new drug therapies brought the crisis under control by the mid-nineties, fashion remains highly aware of its history, with campaigns

above — We need to talk about Kevin: the "Fab Five" dole out some of their famous fashion advice for hopeless straight guys on *The Tonight Show* in 2003 with Kevin Costner.

right — Tomboy style: Katherine Moennig's edgy style inspires straight girls and lesbians alike.

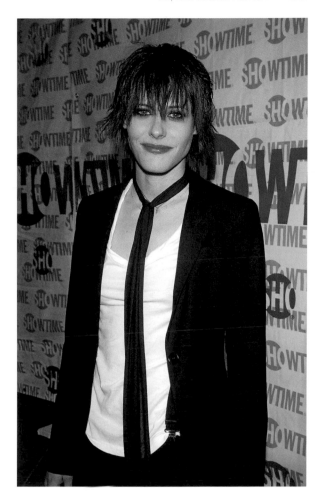

like Fashion Against AIDS continuing to raise awareness.

The dominance of gay fashion designers throughout history is an undeniable fact. The list of names is long: Christian Dior, Yves Saint Laurent, Giorgio Armani, Isaac Mizrahi, and Marc Jacobs are just a sampling. The gender disparity, in fact, has caused significant speculation; the list may be almost entirely gay, but it is also almost entirely male. Lesbian presence in design is very limited, although some credit much of the modern feminine aesthetic to lesbians. In particular, the TV show *Sex and the City* has had a huge influence on modern women's wardrobes, and its lesbian costume designer, Patricia Field, brought a distinctly lesbian aesthetic to the characters: for example, the do-rags and newsboy caps worn by Sarah Jessica Parker easily made their way into straight wardrobes.

In the present, it's difficult to determine a person's orientation simply by the clothes they wear. Some of this is thanks to the rise, in the nineties, of the metrosexual, straight men who had all the style panache of gay men (see "Menswear"). They were the new men, exemplified by the style of David Beckham. Suddenly, it was highly desirable for straight men to resemble gay men as closely as possible—paving the way for later shows like *Queer*

Eye for the Straight Guy. And then there are style icons like the actress Katherine Moennig from *The L Word*, whose cocky tomboy style was imitated by lesbians and straight girls alike.

It's easy to say that much of the way fashion mimics gay and lesbian fashion is thanks to society's growing acceptance of LGBT rights: gay marriage has been legalized in many Western countries, and prominent celebrities and sports stars continue to come out, giving the world an array of gay role models. But there are still places where difference is not respected: the controversial anti-gay laws passed in mid-2013 in Russia are one notorious example. But if history repeats itself, as it so often does, we can be sure of one thing: laws won't prevent gays and lesbians from loving who they want to love, and dressing how they want to dress. And eventually, we'll all be following their lead.

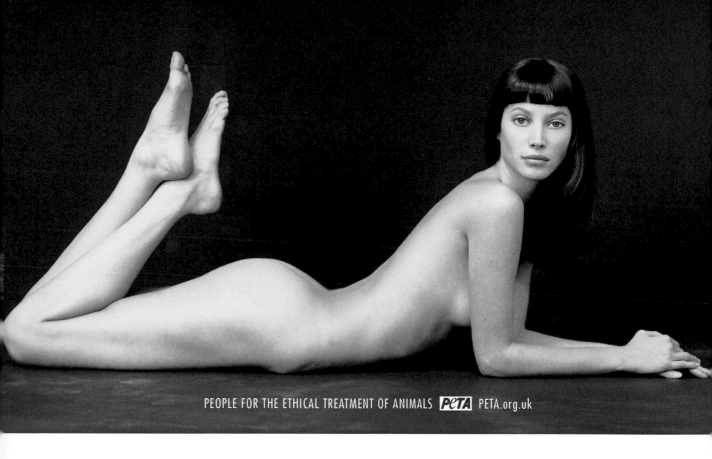

"I'd rather go naked than wear fur."
– Christy Turlington

PEOPLE FOR THE ETHICAL TREATMENT OF ANIMALS **PeTA** PETA.org.uk

above — Since 1990, PETA's sexed-up "I'd Rather Go Naked than Wear Fur" campaign has had an array of fashionable celebrities (like Christy Turlington) pose in the buff for animal rights.

Fashion Ethics

With her artfully spiked black-and-white hair, elbow-length gloves, form-fitting black gown, and flowing fur coat, Cruella de Vil, the villainess from *101 Dalmatians*, is a consummate fashion plate. She's also the embodiment of evil. The sort of person who mercilessly pursues aesthetics at the cost of anything in her path, Cruella wants to make a fur coat out of adorable Dalmatian puppies. There's a reason why she makes such an easy caricature: fashion has long had a problem with ethics. For Cruella to covet fur is an obvious choice: fur has a lengthy history with fashion (particularly high-end), but since it comes from living creatures who sacrifice their lives for its production, wearing it as a fashion statement is riddled with ethical issues. People have worn fur for most of civilization (think of the proverbial caveman wearing a pelt), but by the Middle Ages it had become a status symbol, due to the sumptuary laws that ensured only nobility could wear sought-after furs. But fur really became tied to fashion when the fur trade was established in North America, most of which was based in Canada with the Hudson's Bay Company. The most important pelt, the beaver, was used to create felt hats, popularized by Charles II. Later, fur transitioned from lining coats to being on the outside of them, and by the 1920s, as society indulged itself in the aftermath of World War I, a lush fur coat became a symbol of feminine fashionability and glamour.

But fur's reputation changed in a big way in the 1980s with the growing popularity of the animal rights movement, which charged that animals deserved to live full lives, without suffering. The most notable animal rights organization, People for the Ethical Treatment of Animals (PETA), was founded in early 1980, and immediately took a confrontational, activist approach. Fur was one of their major campaigns, and PETA members became infamous for harassing people wearing fur. One of PETA's best-known campaigns, "I'd Rather Go Naked than Wear Fur," was launched in 1990. Bare-skinned protesters marched with banners bearing this slogan, and celebrities and supermodels posed, naked and provocative, in PETA ads. PETA had their big victory in 1994, after the group occupied Calvin Klein's offices, spray-painting the wall with "kills animals" below the company logo. Klein personally met with the group, and then announced to the world that he would stop producing furs. A number of other designers followed suit.

By 1996, animal rights activists had a new foe: *Vogue* editor Anna Wintour, who declared her affection for fur in that year's September issue. Soon after,

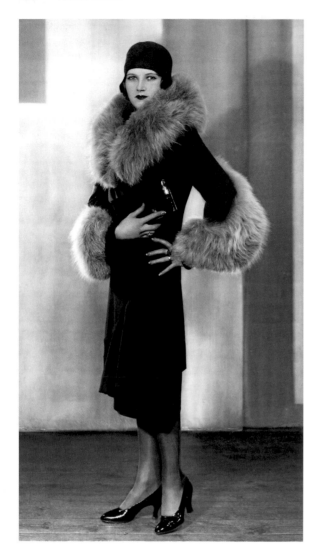

rose in the wake of the Industrial Revolution, when most garment production took place in the factories of London and New York. Factory owners tried to get as much out of their workers as possible, and criticism of sweatshops appeared as early as 1850. The big event that galvanized the anti-sweatshop movement was a tragic one: the Triangle Shirtwaist Factory fire, which broke out in New York's Greenwich Village in 1911. Killing 146 garment workers, it still ranks as one of the city's deadliest disasters, and it brought much attention to factory conditions. Resulting labor laws improved factory conditions in developed countries throughout the twentieth century, but sweatshops do still exist, even in New York and London.

By the nineties, globalization had pushed most gar-

a protestor threw a dead raccoon onto her plate at the Four Seasons restaurant. But Wintour led the zeitgeist, and since the nineties, fur has seen a resurgence, also due to the marketing efforts of the fur industry, which has funded the use of fur in design. PETA, nonetheless, soldiers on—and the ethical quagmire has gotten worse in recent years, as the more unregulated Chinese fur market has been revealed to use dog and cat fur, paying little heed to treating animals humanely.

It's not only animals that suffer for fashion; often, people do too, particularly those who work in the overcrowded and unsafe sweatshops that help maintain our supply of cheap clothing. Sweatshops

left — Speakeasies, flappers, and fur: in the Roaring Twenties a fur coat was a sure sign of a classy dame.

right — The devil wears fur: Anna Wintour (shown here in 2010) raises the hackles of animal rights advocates with her pro-fur stance.

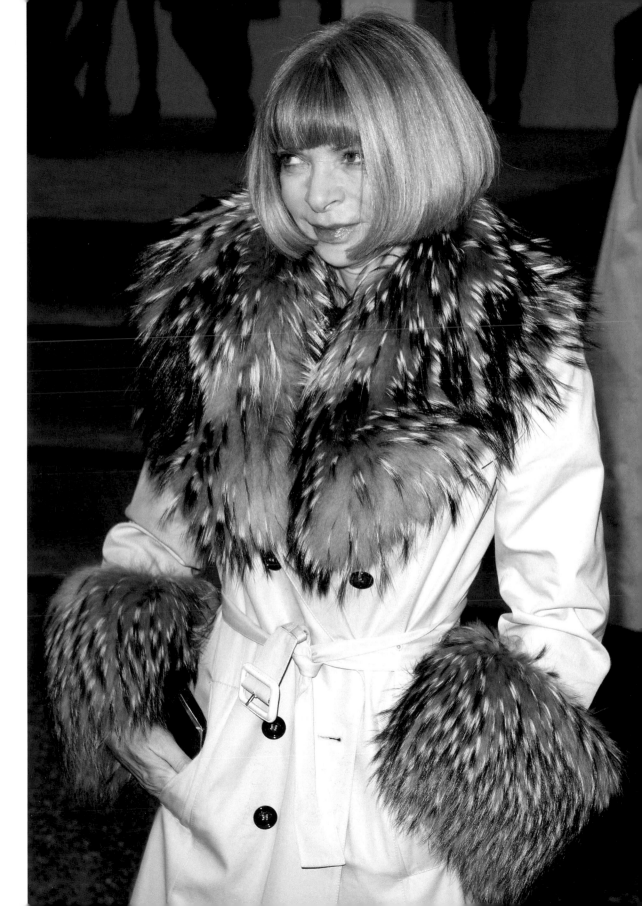

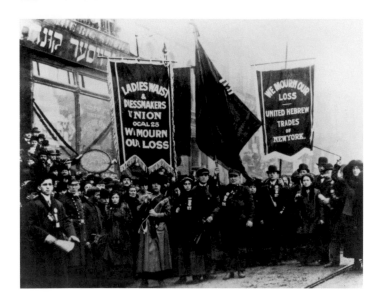

ment production offshore to places such as China, where production was jaw-droppingly cheap—but also difficult to regulate. The exploitation of workers in foreign countries became a new focus for activists, and the issue was helped into mainstream consciousness by Naomi Klein's book *No Logo* (2000), which highlighted the labor practices of apparel producers like Gap and Nike. All the bad press pushed these companies to adopt more ethically sound production practices.

The ethically conscious ethos of the new millennium also provided the perfect environment for the growth of American Apparel, which uses "sweatshop free" as a marketing catchphrase for its trendy cotton basics. Opening its first factory in Los Angeles in 1997, the vertically integrated company gives its workers what it considers a living wage, health care, regular hours, and other benefits. Today, it operates the largest clothing factory in North America—though American Apparel has recently gone through some financial struggles, which have as much to do with the company's rapid retail expansion as with the lecherous public persona of its founder, Canadian Dov Charney.

The ethical manufacturing practices of companies like American Apparel ensure that their products will never be cheap, making it tough for them to compete with fast fashion, which fills most closets today. Pioneered by Spanish retailer Zara, fast fashion offers year-round new styles copied from runway looks at rock-bottom prices, which only works when a company sells high volumes at a low profit margin. With its dependence on ultralow manufacturing costs, fast fashion has increased the competition for offshore production. By the second decade of the twenty-first century, China's expanding economy and growing standard of living had pushed costs higher there. This led companies to pursue manufacturing in countries such as Bangladesh, whose less-regulated factories regularly experience news-making disasters, such as the deadly Rana Plaza factory collapse in April 2013, which killed more than 1,100 people.

Fashion, with its cyclical trends and mass consump-

above — In the wake of the devastating Triangle Shirtwaist Factory fire, garment workers unionized and demanded better working conditions.

right — Sweatshop free, with a dash of sleaze: American Apparel CEO Dov Charney is equally known for pursuing ethical working conditions—and his own peccadilloes.

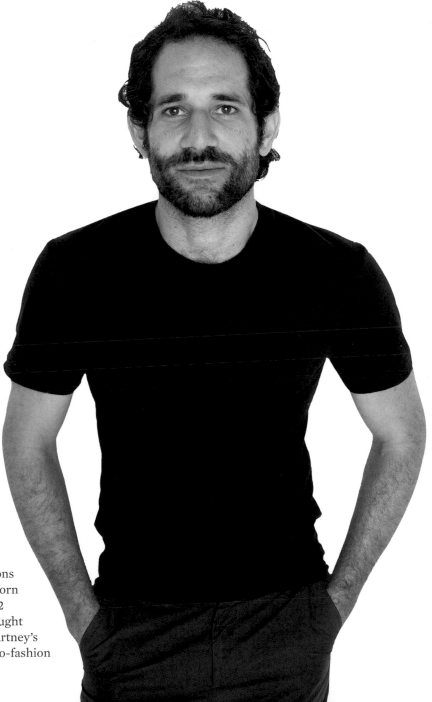

tion, is inherently wasteful—it uses up resources and pollutes the earth, often for frivolous reasons. It is a truth that inspired the sustainable fashion movement, which aspires to be ecofriendly and socially responsible. One of the earliest proponents of ecofriendly fashion was English designer Katharine Hamnett, best known for her political slogan T-shirts of the eighties. Hamnett named her 1989 collection "Clean Up or Die" after discovering the effects of pesticide poisoning on cotton farmers. From that point, the designer lobbied for fair-trade, organic cotton in clothing production.

Despite edgy designers like Hamnett, sustainable fashion suffered for many years from associations with the shapeless hemp clothing worn by some hippies. It wasn't until 2002 that ethical fashion became truly sought after with the launch of Stella McCartney's eponymous label, the first luxury eco-fashion

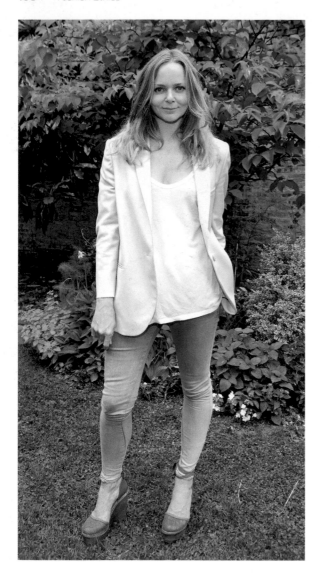

line. As a vegetarian, McCartney makes clothing that is fur and leather free. Not all of her clothing is ecofriendly, but she makes a conscious effort to use organic or recycled fabrics—the designer asserts that "something is better than nothing."

After McCartney's success, other high-end eco-fashion lines popped up, like Loomstate, which debuted in 2004 as the first luxury organic denim line, and EDUN, founded in 2005 by Ali Hewson and her husband, U2's Bono, to promote fair trade with Africa. Despite this progress, some say that eco-fashion itself is a farce, just an example of "green-washing": when people consume fashion at high volumes, it's inherently wasteful, no matter whether the fabric is organic.

Beyond manufacturing, fashion is also criticized for its influence on women's (and, to a smaller but growing degree, men's) body image. While fashion's focus has historically been on beauty rather than the "average woman," the definition of beauty has changed drastically since the twentieth century: today's extra-skinny models are often blamed for widespread body issues and eating disorders.

above — Green goddess: lifelong vegetarian Stella McCartney (photographed here in 2011) succeeded in making eco-chic truly fashionable.

right — Far from frumpy, McCartney's eco-conscious clothing, shown here at the Fashion Institute of Technology, fashionably captures sustainability's zeitgeist.

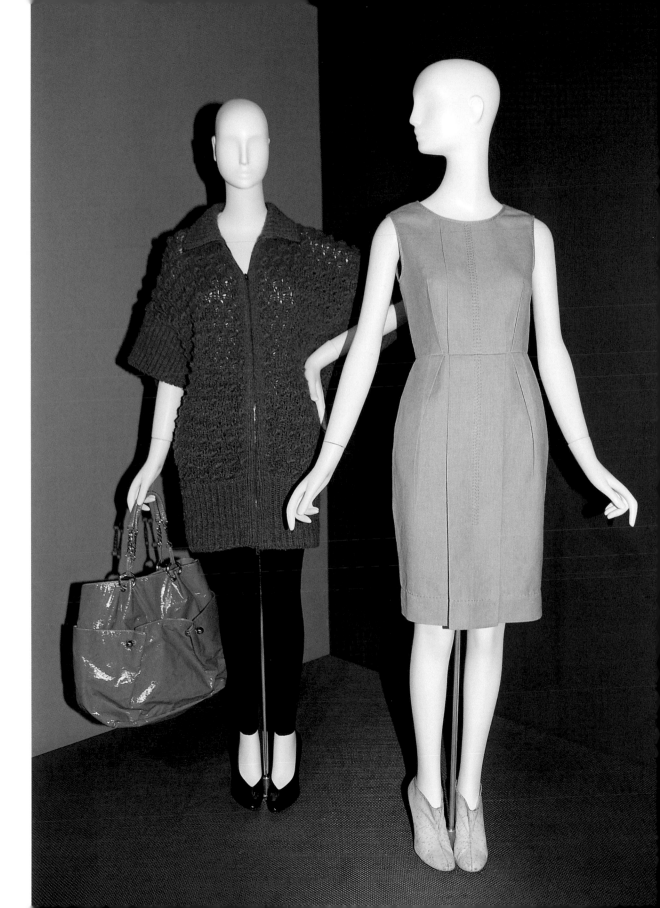

Some of this is due to Photoshopping, which came under great scrutiny in 2009 for producing images of women that were anatomically impossible (see "Fashion Photography"). In 2009, *Glamour* responded by running an unretouched photo of a size 12–14 model, Lizzie Miller, to overwhelming reader response. In 2010, other fashion magazines went against the ultra-skinny trend, running fashion stories with plus-size models, such as *V* magazine's "Size" issue. But it was hardly a sea change. In 2012, controversy emerged when a fourteen-year-old girl petitioned *Seventeen* magazine to limit Photoshopping; the magazine responded, agreeing to "Never change girls' body shapes or faces," an oblique statement that left the magazine's intent vague. Today, Photoshopping remains an everyday practice.

But the problems don't just exist in photography. Beginning with the "heroin chic" waifs of the nineties like Kate Moss (see "Fashion Models"), models themselves have become thinner, often unhealthily so. In response, the Council of Fashion Designers of America (in association with *Vogue*) launched the Health Initiative in 2007, setting minimum age limits for models and mandating against hiring models with eating disorders. Yet little has changed: in July 2013, the *Guardian* published an exposé by former *Vogue* Australia editor Kirstie Clements about the diminishing size of models—some of whom, she

asserts, do things as dramatic as eating tissues or going on an IV drip to avoid gaining weight—striving for an ideal neither healthy nor realistic for most women. She puts partial blame on designers themselves, who send samples in a size 0 that even many naturally lithe models cannot fit into.

Many of these ethical issues are influenced every day by the millions of consumers who buy fashion. Fashion isn't just about the way we look—on a greater scale, it affects the lives of people around the world, animals, and the earth itself. It's possible to choose not to wear fur (or to wear faux fur) to support animal rights, to choose to buy products manufactured by companies who use ethical factories, and to reduce our environmental impact by buying a limited number of quality pieces rather than dozens of the latest trends. Magazines may present us with emaciated models, but we don't have to buy the magazines, or the clothes, if we don't like what we see. Even Cruella de Vil had a choice—she just chose to be evil.

right — Nothing artificial: *Glamour*'s 2009 shot of an unretouched Lizzie Miller, a size 12–14 model, was embraced by readers for its refreshingly real beauty.

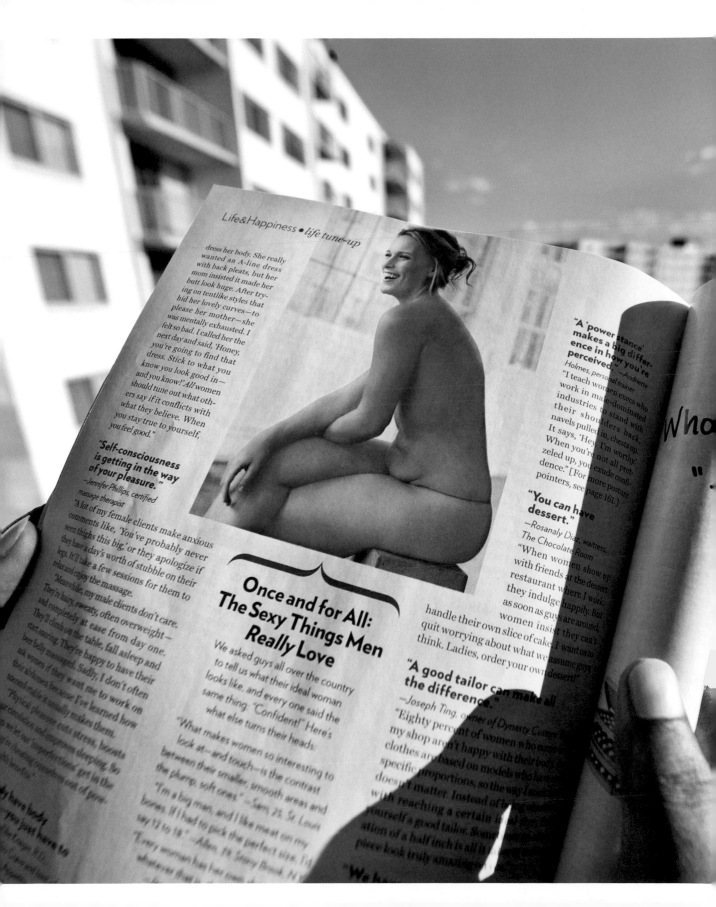

dress her body. She really wanted an A-line dress with back pleats, but her mom insisted it made her butt look huge. After trying on tentlike styles that hid her lovely curves—to please her mother—she was mentally exhausted. I felt so bad. I called her the next day and said, 'Honey, you're going to find that dress. Stick to what you know you look good in—and you know!' All women should tune out what others say if it conflicts with what they believe. When you stay true to yourself, you feel good."

"Self-consciousness is getting in the way of your pleasure."
—*Jennifer Phillips, certified massage therapist*

"A lot of my female clients make anxious comments like, 'You've probably never seen thighs this big,' or they apologize if they have a day's worth of stubble on their legs. It'll take a few sessions for them to relax and enjoy the massage.

"Meanwhile, my male clients don't care. They're hairy, sweaty, often overweight—and completely at ease from day one. They'll climb on the table, fall asleep and start snoring. They're happy to have their beer belly massaged. Sadly, I don't often ask women if they want me to work on their abdomen because I've learned how uncomfortable it usually makes them.

"Physical pleasure cuts stress, boosts circulation and improves sleep. So we do ourselves a big disservice when we let our imperfections get in the way of feeling good."

[obscured by shadow]

Once and for All: The Sexy Things Men Really Love

We asked guys all over the country to tell us what their ideal woman looks like, and every one said the same thing: "Confident!" Here's what else turns their heads:

"What makes women so interesting to look at—and touch—is the contrast between their smaller, smooth areas and the plump, soft ones." —*Sam 23, St. Louis*

"I'm a big man, and I like meat on my bones. If I had to pick the perfect size, I'd say 12 to 14." —*Allen 19, Stony Brook, N.Y.*

"Every woman has her own [obscured]

"A 'power stance' makes a big difference in how you're perceived."
—*Andriette Holmes, personal trainer*

"I teach women execs who work in male-dominated industries to stand with their shoulders back, navels pulled in, chests up. It says, 'Hey, I'm worthy.' When you're not all pretzeled up, you exude confidence." [For more posture pointers, see page 161.]

"You can have dessert."
—*Rosanaly Diaz, waitress, The Chocolate Room*

"When women show up with friends at the dessert restaurant where I work, they indulge happily. But as soon as guys are around, women insist they can't handle their own slice of cake! I want us to quit worrying about what we assume guys think. Ladies, order your own dessert!"

"A good tailor can make all the difference."
—*Joseph Ting, owner of Dynasty Custom*

"Eighty percent of women who come to my shop aren't happy with their body. Clothes are based on models who have specific proportions, so the way [obscured] doesn't matter. Instead of [obscured] with reaching a certain [obscured] yourself a good tailor. Sometimes [obscured] ation of a half inch is all it [obscured] piece look truly amazing [obscured]

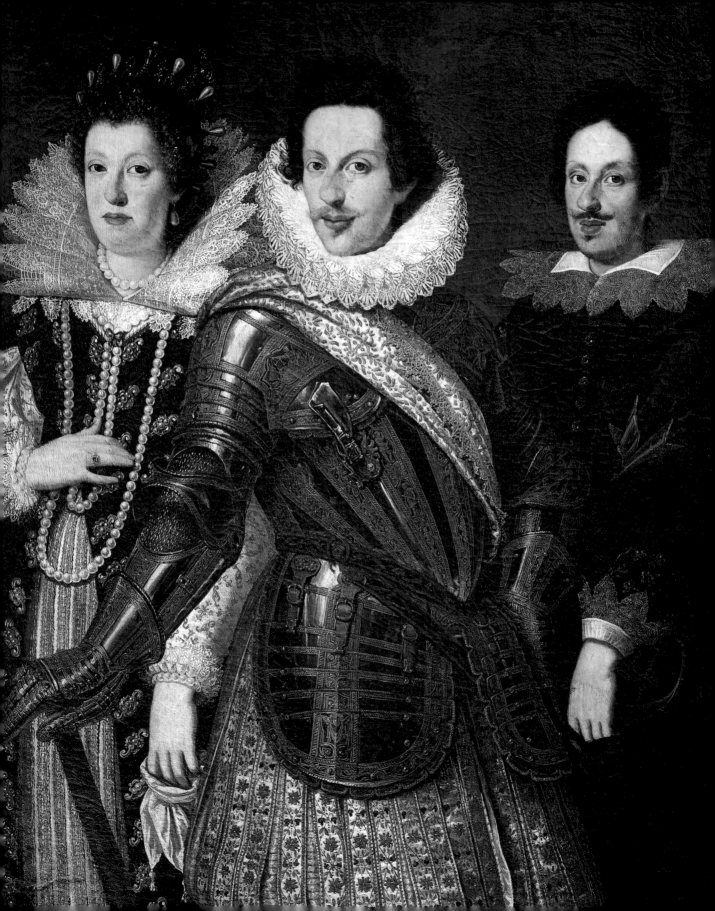

Fashion Capitals

The very word "Paris" drips fashion. But there's a reason why the effortlessly stylish Parisian woman, quaffing red wine at sidewalk cafés, haunts our dreams of the French capital: it is because she's real. For hundreds of years, Paris has been a bona fide fashion city, dictating to the rest of the world how to dress well. But it hasn't always been that way. And today, Paris is in the company of other fashion cities, which routinely challenge its claim to style supremacy: London, New York and Milan.

To truly be a fashion capital, a city needs to tick off a few boxes: it requires fashion infrastructure (the business and the artisans that support the creation of fashion), it needs a thriving design scene, and it must exert international influence. Often, influence is tied to a city's overall power and economic muscle, and it always involves a city being a leading cultural hub. Many cities in the world make clothes, but most of those cities don't lead style around the globe. That's why fashion capitals are special. The first fashion capitals were in Italy, a direct result of that country's place at the heart of the Renaissance. Italy was known for its textiles, and the fashions worn by powerful families such as the Medicis influenced fashion across Europe. As the seat of the Medicis' power, Florence was the pinnacle of Renaissance style.

After the Medicis fell from power, Spanish fashions came into the fore, all severe blacks and formality. But those conservative fashions fell away with the rise of Paris. Paris's roots in clothing manufacture go back a long way, but its ascendance to fashion capital began under the reign of Louis XIV, the Sun King (see "Royal Fashion"). Louis flaunted his belief in his divine right to power through fashion, and dressed both himself and his court in truly decadent fashion. One of the keys to Paris's status as a fashion capital was (and still is) the French government's recognition of the importance of fashion to the French economy. As early as the seventeenth century, under Louis's rule, the French government began implementing measures to support the fashion business. In this environment, small ateliers (dressmakers, tailors, mercers, milliners) flourished across Paris to as part of the growing industry.

left — Wealthy and well dressed, the Medicis made Florence a fashion hub. This seventeenth-century portrait shows Cosimo II de Medici with his wife Maria Maddalena and his son Francesco.

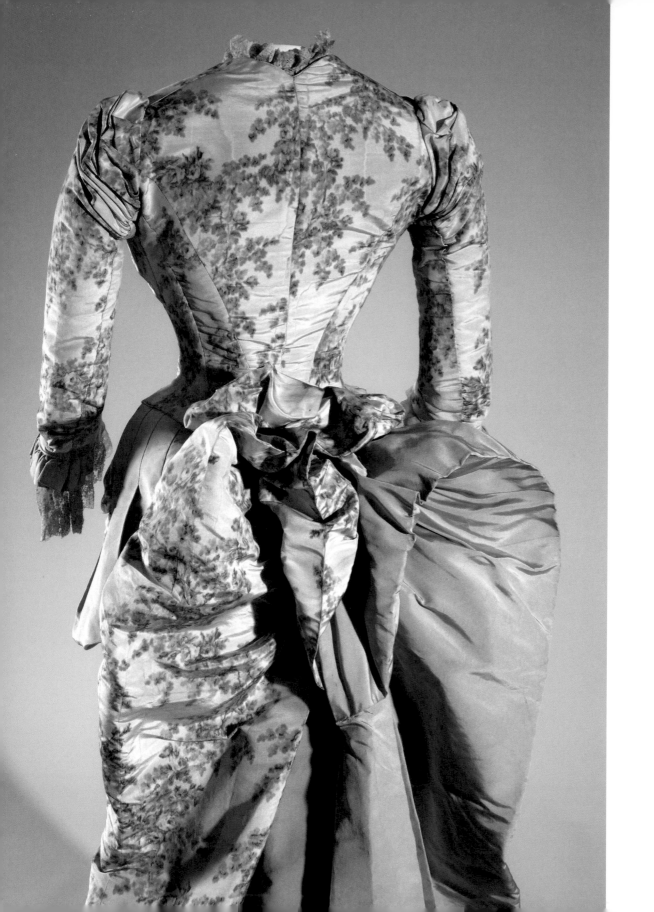

This set the stage for one of history's most influential fashion figures, Marie Antoinette, who used style (often provocative, sometimes controversial) in a fierce bid to secure her own power. A supreme manipulator of public opinion through fashion, Marie Antoinette began debuting her styles in Paris rather than in court at Versailles, opening herself up to imitators among the city's fashionable women. At the same time, she allowed her designers in Paris to sell things designed for her to the public at large. With Marie Antoinette setting fashions, Paris leaping upon them immediately, and the rest of Europe lusting after them in rapid succession, Paris was the indisputable center of all fashion.

But the city truly came into its own in the nineteenth century, when Charles Worth opened up what was to become the first couture business (see "Couture"). Worth's innovation was to impose his creative vision on his clients, rather than taking their direction—in turn making his own name as an artist.

left — Worthy beginnings: Charles Frederick Worth brought couture to Paris, giving the city the first claim on high-end made-to-measure fashion. Shown here is a House of Worth dress from 1883.

Worth's luxurious made-to-measure fashions set the bar for how the wealthiest people in France and around the world should dress. His clients included people like Empress Eugénie and Sarah Bernhardt, and his dresses cost a small fortune. His startling success brought on a massive wave of couture designers that surged until the 1960s: Paul Poiret, Chanel, and Dior all owe their business model to his pioneering ways.

Paris's fashion dominance came to a halt during World War II, during Paris's great trauma under the occupation of the Nazis. Normal life was on hold for most Parisians during this time. Paris managed to resist having its fashion business relocated wholesale to Vienna or Berlin due to the actions of Lucien Lelong, who led the organizational body that advocated for couture (the Chambre syndicale de la haute couture)—but while fashion design still took place in the city, it wasn't like it was before the war. Many designers fled, and Paris was largely cut off from the rest of the fashion universe; nobody wanted to travel to the city to view collections. And so New York stepped up to bat.

Up to this point, New York hadn't taken a role in global fashion leadership, although many designers had found success in the city, of a quiet sort. New York had hidden its creativity behind imitations

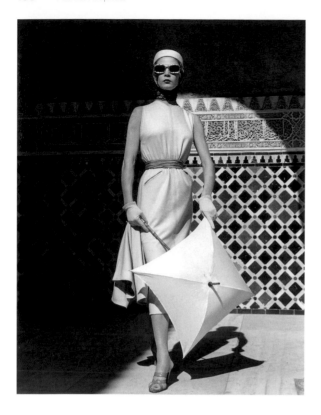

of Paris. Department stores would make copies of designs from the French capital, and sometimes designers would even pass off their own designs as Parisian labels. War-imposed shortages of Paris fashions, of course, meant that New York designers needed to stand behind their own ideas. Fashion magazines began to cover American designs, and in an effort to boost the industry, a publicist named Eleanor Lambert launched the very first fashion week in 1943 (called "Press Week"). Designers like Claire McCardell and Charles James vaulted into recognition, and Mainbocher, an American couturier who had made his name in Paris, flourished anew in New York in 1940 after fleeing the occupation. But Paris wasn't done for good; the city's fashion industry did recover after the war, and quite dramatically, with Dior's New Look. The ultrafeminine New Look took the world by storm, and the fashion media flocked to cover the city in its new ascendance. But in the sixties, it was time for London to dust off the cobwebs. London had long been a bit of a player, and was widely known for its tailoring. But its big fashion moment came when youth culture exploded

in the city's streets, and style began to be influenced by the radically youthful clothing worn by subcultures like the mods and rockers (see "Fashion Subcultures"). Suddenly, couture began to seem old and stuffy, and people swarmed to buy clothes from the likes of Mary Quant (who became known for her miniskirts and hot pants) and Biba; London stayed strong until the hippie movement picked up speed, and the image of Swinging London dissipated—though the city was revived by the punk ethos of Vivienne Westwood in the seventies.

In the seventies, one of the oldest fashion capitals reemerged: Milan. Italian fashion in general experienced success due to the post-World War II economic regeneration of Italy: Florence captured the interest of fashionistas with its boutique fashions, for a period, and Rome's couture garnered some

above — Designers like Claire McCardell, whose informal, ready-to-wear designs rejected the stiffness of Parisian couture, put New York on the map.

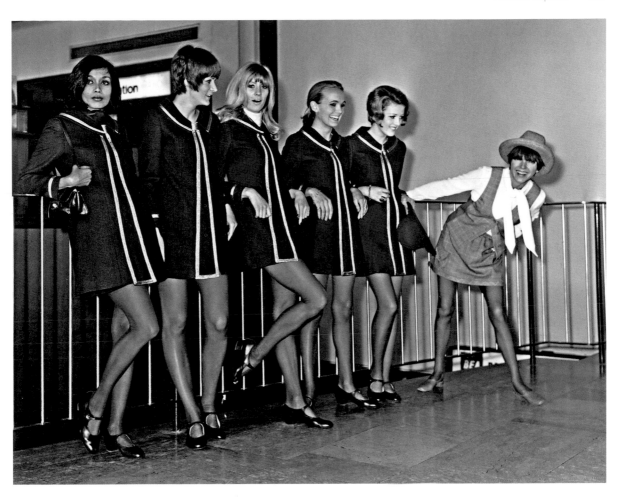

attention. But the rising popularity of ready-to-wear (launched into prominence in Paris by Yves Saint Laurent) led to the rise and eventual dominance of Milan. It was Milanese designers who perfected the image of luxury ready-to-wear. Designers like Armani and Versace brought Italian cool to the fore, and Milan has remained a recognized hub for fashion ever since. At the same time, New York was also proving its mettle in the ready-to-wear market, with designers like Calvin Klein and Ralph Lauren (see "Ready-to-Wear and Mass Fashion").

above — The London look goes international: here, Mary Quant and her models pose at Heathrow before a continental fashion tour in 1968.

Paris, Milan, London, New York: since the seventies, that's been the mantra. Tokyo sometimes makes the list, too—but while street fashions in the Japanese capital are influential (in particular, the colorful street styles of the Harajuku district have captured international imaginations), the biggest, most influential Japanese designers have found fame working in other cities, usually Paris (see "Global Fashion"). Yohji Yamamoto, for example, made his name in Paris in the eighties; Rei Kawakubo began in Tokyo but eventually also focused her efforts in Paris during the same decade; and Kenzo had already burst onto the fashion scene in Paris in the seventies. And then there's Antwerp, certainly a fashion city of note. The Belgian city isn't really a full-fledged fashion capital; it's too reliant on the fashion infrastructure of other cities, mostly Paris, to claim that prize.

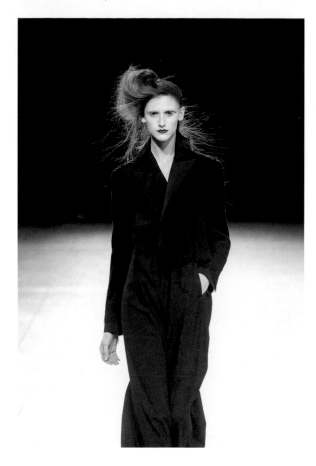

But the prominence of the avant-garde Antwerp Six (Walter Van Beirendonck, Ann Demeulemeester, Dries Van Noten, Dirk Van Saene, Dirk Bikkembergs and Marina Yee) as well as Martin Margiela (who relocated to Paris) put it on the map.

Recently, attention has been lavished, once again, on London; the city is home to the still showstopping Alexander McQueen (now under Sarah Burton) and a raft of other hot designers like Stella McCartney and Tom Ford. Not to mention the media sensation that is Kate Middleton, whose high/low fashion choices have inspired millions. Power, economic muscle, and a hot design scene: London ticks off all those boxes for reigning fashion capital.

Over the years, the Big Four fashion cities have moved up and down the ranks, but their reputations are cemented. Though who's ranking as number one often changes (and varies depending on who you ask), they all reliably place. These cities all have history, healthy economies, and an established fashion culture on their side. But as the global economy shifts, we'll doubtless see some challengers. Fashion weeks have popped up around the globe, and though they may not all be taken seriously, one day we may see a real contender among the likes of Berlin, Istanbul, São Paulo, Mumbai—or some pleasantly unexpected other.

above — Fashion provocateur Yohji Yamamoto is known for pairing the avant-garde with traditional Japanese aesthetics. Here, a model shows off one of his ready-to-wear designs in Paris in 2009.

right — Beautiful as ever, British designer Sarah Burton's designs continue the legacy of Alexander McQueen. Shown here is a look from the Fall/Winter 2012–13 ready-to-wear collection.

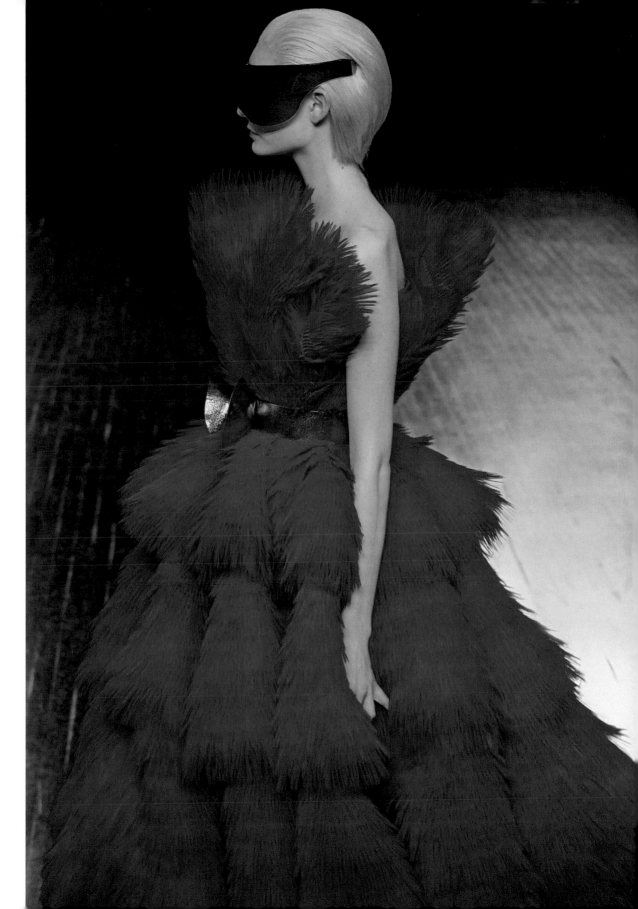

Global Fashion

ashion Week Internationale, a VICE web series hosted by a fearless ex-model turned journalist named Charlet Duboc, takes viewers backstage for fashion weeks in far-flung, sometimes dangerous locales: Islamabad, Tel Aviv, Medellin, and Lagos are just a few. Gritty and revealing, the show offers a glimpse of the passion felt by people around the globe for expressing themselves through style. And it's true: there's more to fashion than just what's on offer from Western designers—though most international fashion has yet to break through on a global scale.

When it comes to non-Western fashion, Japan is in a category by itself. Daring and avant-garde, its influence on worldwide style over the last few decades has been immense. It all began when Japan was first exposed to Western fashion during the radical modernization of the Meiji period, which lasted from 1868 to 1912 and triggered Japan's own industrial revolution. By the end of the Meiji period, the Japanese wore Western fashions as a symbol of their new modernity and economic prosperity, while expanding trade inspired the West's interest in Japanese aesthetics (a trend called Japonisme). Japan faced further exposure to Western styles in the aftermath of World War II, when America had a heavy hand in the country's postwar administration.

In postwar Japan, youth culture (see "Fashion Sub-cultures") and ready-to-wear clothing thrived, and Japanese street style began to appear. This environment proved the perfect breeding ground for the new wave of Japanese fashion designers. First among these was Kenzo Takada. Takada moved to Paris in 1964 to establish himself in the world of fashion—which was to be the path of most Japanese designers in his wake, due to the lack of fashion infrastructure within the country (see "Fashion Capitals"). Kenzo founded the House of Kenzo in 1970, and his first store, Jungle Jap, made waves with its colorful, original designs. Other successful designers followed during the seventies, notably Issey Miyake, who later became known for his inventive pleating, and Hanae Mori, the first Asian woman inducted into the Fédération française de la couture.

While the Japanese fashion of the seventies made remarkable headway in the Paris fashion scene,

right — Indian heat: Manish Arora became known as "the John Galliano of India" for his wild fashions. Shown here is a design from his Fall/Winter 2012–13 collection.

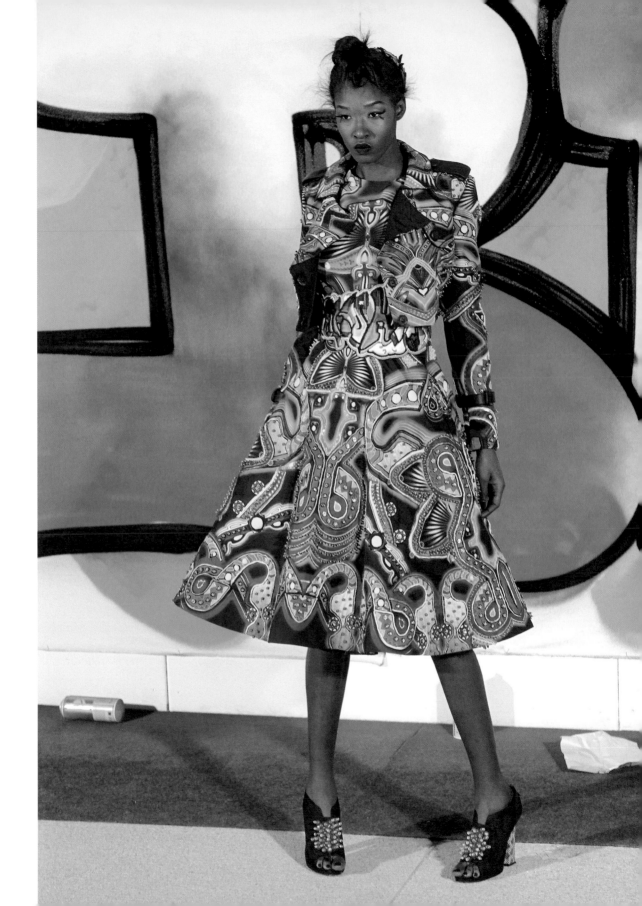

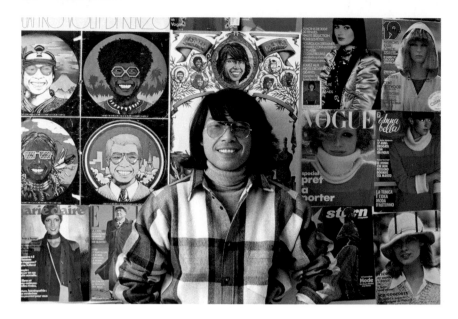

what came in the eighties was truly revolutionary. Two designers in particular were the genesis of what was to be a radical shift in aesthetics: Rei Kawakubo, with her line Comme des Garçons, and Yohji Yamamoto. Both showed in Paris in 1981, shocking and provoking the fashion world with their blatant disregard for anything fitted or pretty in pursuit of something altogether more artistic. Both designers steeped their work in shades of black and used uneven, torn, deconstructed shapes that many deemed apocalyptic. Yamamoto's and Kawakubo's influence can be seen in some of the fashions of the grunge era, as well as in the work of the avant-garde Belgian designers like Ann Demeulemeester, Dries Van Noten, and Martin Margiela. Both Kawakubo and Yamamoto continue to reliably produce edgy, sometimes shocking fashions, while newer designers like Junya Watanabe (Kawakubo's protégé) experiment in other ways; Watanabe is a virtuoso with technical fabrics.

At the same time as Japanese couture was taking over the West, Tokyo's street style was coming into full bloom. Starting in 1977 and ending in 1998, the area around Tokyo's Harajuku Station was pedestrianized, the perfect place for youths to hang out and flaunt inventive fashions. By the nineties, Tokyo had an international reputation for its wild street styles,

and there were several different sartorial subsets, including (but far from limited to) manga-influenced styles, cosplay (costume play), and the gothic Lolita, which featured little-girl cute outfits in funereal black. The worship of *kawaii*, or cuteness, is an enduring feature of Japanese street style. Some Japanese designers have translated Harajuku street fashion into higher-end style, most notably Jun Takahashi with his label Undercover, while Nigo's coveted line A Bathing Ape concentrates on more casual streetwear.

Fashion is typically fueled by a growing economy—the birth of the Western and Japanese fashion industries were both the result of the Industrial Revolution (see "Couture"). Perhaps unsurprisingly, there's a lot of promise in the nascent fashion industries

above — Kenzo Takada, pictured here during his "Jungle Jap" phase in 1975, was the first of a succession of Japanese designers to make waves in the fashion world.

right — The enigmatic queen of anti-fashion, Rei Kawakubo designs avant-garde, deconstructed looks for her label Comme des Garçons, like this one from her Fall/Winter 2004–05 collection.

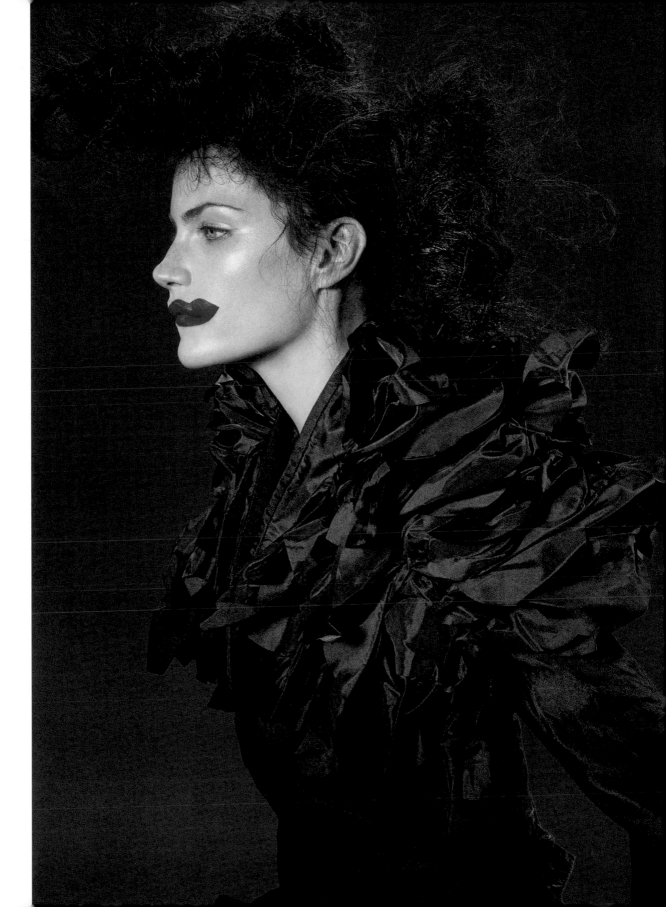

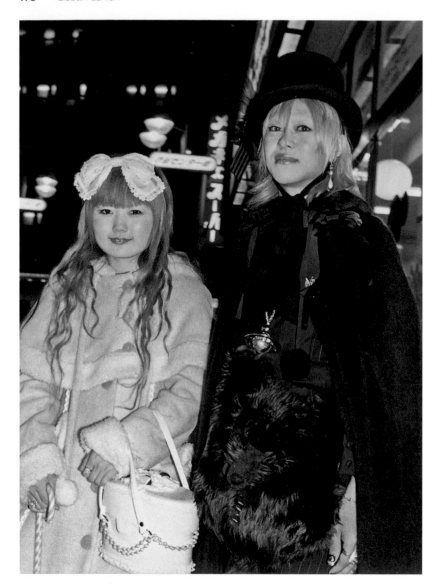

of today's emerging economies, which are encapsulated by the convenient acronym BRICS: Brazil, Russia, India, China, and South Africa (though African fashion is by no means limited to the continent's southernmost point).

Brazil evokes nothing more strongly than frolicking on a beach with a caipirinha, and the country has long been associated with swimwear and beach apparel; perhaps its best-known brand is Havaianas, colorful flip-flops that first became popular in 1962. But as the country has grown more prosperous, it has yearned to brush off a bit of the sand. As international luxury brands have proliferated in the shopping districts of Rio de Janeiro and São Paulo, the country has tried to escape its reputation for simple, sunny attire: Gloria Coelho and Alexandre Herchcovitch are good examples of Brazil's growingly sophisticated edge.

above — So *kawaii*: in this photo, two Tokyo teenagers show off the "Pink Lolita" style and the "Elegant Gothic Aristocrat" look.

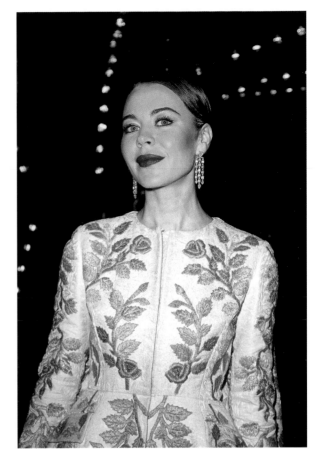

While Brazil bucks tradition, India, for the most part, embraces it. Designer saris are big business, and the ever-growing fashion industry is heavily influenced by the glitz and glamour of Bollywood: big-name designer Manish Malhotra caters largely to the Bollywood crowd, and his looks are decadent and steeped in Indian history. One designer to break through into the global market is Manish Arora, who has been nicknamed the "John Galliano of India" for his colorful, over-the-top designs that integrate traditional Indian beading and embroidery. Arora's international acclaim led to a brief role as creative director for Paco Rabanne between 2011 and 2012. Despite its recent hunger for designer goods, China's homegrown fashion scene is still growing slowly. China was, of course, for many years the hub of world clothing manufacture (Bangladesh is poised, these days, to take its place; see "Fashion Ethics")— but despite the in-depth knowledge of how to cut and sew complex fashions, most design has always

been done in other countries. In the last few years, however, some promising designers have started to emerge, like Qiu Hao, who won the prestigious Woolmark Prize in 2008.

Russia's domestic design scene remains small, but its influence on global fashion trends has spiked sharply in recent years as the country's rich have become dramatically wealthier. Russia's moneyed fashion lovers have started buying up couture in jaw-dropping quantities, and savvy designers have begun to pander to their tastes. Some of these rich Russians have become style stars in their own right, such as Ulyana Sergeenko—a much-photographed Russian billionaire's wife who recently started her own eponymous couture label, which debuted in Paris in 2012.

Africa's influence extends far beyond South Africa; the continent has long been a source of inspiration to many designers, though the influence of African-born designers isn't as acknowledged. And yet, two

above — Billionaire Girls' Club: Ulyana Sergeenko has successfully transitioned from couture customer to couturier, successfully showing her collections in Paris since 2012. She's photographed here in October 2013 at Paris Fashion Week.

Northern African designers are verified fashion royalty: Yves Saint Laurent (born in Algeria) and Azzedine Alaïa (born in Tunisia). The two sometimes display evidence of their birth in their designs, such as YSL's African collection of 1967 and Safari jacket of 1968, and Alaïa's African-inspired sandals of 2010. But as Africa becomes more prosperous, it is beginning to move beyond the influence of these two heavyweights. One of the first of the new African designers was Malian Lamine Badian Kouyaté, whose line Xuly Bët shook things up with its colorful punk/African fashions in the nineties and was rewarded with an ANDAM Award in 1996. A more recent example is Nigerian Amaka Osakwe, whose line, Maki Oh, uses hand-dyed African textiles to create refined, feminine dresses and skirts that have been seen on people like Solange Knowles and Michelle Obama. Designers like Osakwe have piqued significant interest in the continent's fashion industry, spurring events like Africa Fashion Week, which has taken place in London since 2011, and fashion magazine *Arise*, which documents African fashion.

An interesting sidebar on the burgeoning African design scene is the ongoing subculture of the Congolese *sapeurs*, the dandies of Africa. The existence of sapeurs (whose name comes from the acronym SAPE: La Société des ambianceurs et des personnes élégantes) can be traced to France's colonial influence in the early twentieth century, when residents of the Congo were exposed to Parisian fashion. Mostly working-class residents of Brazzaville and Kinshasa, sapeurs invest shocking quantities of money into tailored suits from well-known Parisian designers, often in bright colors, pairing them with smartly coordinated hats, ties, and pocket squares: this peacocking elevates their lives above the squalor and poverty of their homeland. Their styles have become so known worldwide that the sapeurs no longer simply take inspiration from couture, but rather inspire it: mostly notably, Paul Smith's 2010 women's collection mimicked the looks worn by many of the sapeurs documented in the book *Gentlemen of Bacongo* by photographer Daniele Tamagni.

There are many more countries that would love to show off their designs on the world stage, as revealed by the growing number of international fashion weeks (*Fashion Week Internationale* just captures a handful of these). A quick Google search reveals long lists of fashion weeks happening every month of the year in places as diverse as Dar Es Salaam, Kiev, Fiji, and Goa. Whether they're recognized abroad or just domestically, these fashion weeks are evidence that even in a world dominated by Western fashion, people want to flaunt their own style, whatever its roots may be.

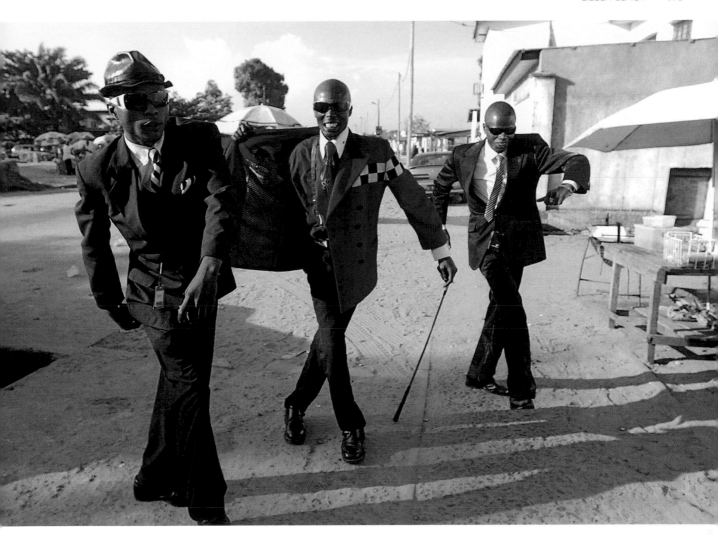

above — The dandies of Africa, sapeurs flaunt their style in
the streets of the Congo. Shown here is a trio of sapeurs in
Kinshasa in 2010.

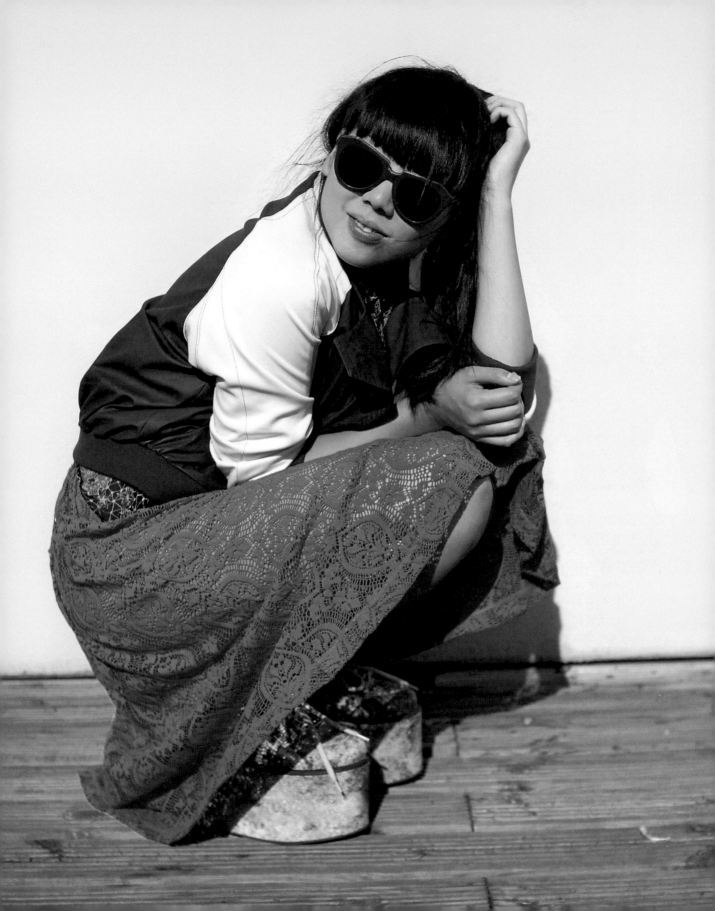

Fashion and the Internet

In 2009, some grumpy fashion editors at Paris Fashion Week had a complaint: a giant bow was blocking their view at Dior's runway show. To show their displeasure, they tweeted about it, and the image made the rounds on the internet. It wasn't simply the bow itself that was bugging them, but also who was wearing it: Tavi Gevinson, only thirteen years old, and also a blogger.

The internet has changed the fashion industry in many ways, one of the most noticeable being how it has democratized and made it accessible to everyone, even teenagers in their suburban bedrooms. Nothing represents the average person more than bloggers, those self-appointed experts who can publish their opinions to the world while wearing pajamas, if that's what they choose. Making a mark in fashion no longer requires a degree in journalism or a sought-after position at a fashion magazine—all any blogger needs is an internet connection.

People have been writing about fashion on the internet for a long time—on the early, text-based internet, so-called "newsgroups" were the primary discussion forums, and one called alt.fashion became popular in the early nineties. Newsgroups like alt.fashion paved the way for later, more interactive sites like *The Fashion Spot*, which boasted discussion forums and options for people to share photos of their own personal style.

Blogging itself started to become popular around 1999; easy-to-use platforms such as LiveJournal and Blogger launched that year, while some of the first documented fashion blogs appeared around 2002. One early blog of note was *A Shaded View on Fashion*, created in 2005 by fashion journalist Diane Pernet. *ASVOF* offered an insider perspective on the fashion industry featuring interviews, short films, and drawings. But the blog that really changed everything was *The Sartorialist*. Launched in 2005 by Scott Schuman, who had quit his day job to care for his daughter, the site compelled audiences with the stylish informality of its subjects: Schuman photographed regular people (who just happened to be very well dressed) going about their day-to-day activities. Schuman certainly didn't invent the idea of street style—many photographers had been capturing it for years, most notably Bill Cunningham for the *New York Times* beginning in the seventies. But *The Sartorialist* made it work online.

left — Rising to the top: fashion blogger Susie Bubble found fame documenting her own personal style.

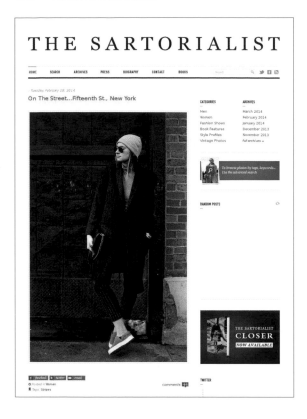

The beauty of online street-style blogs was that people sitting at home could easily imagine themselves in the photos; after all, the photographic subjects typically weren't models, but people like themselves. Around the same time as *The Sartorialist*, a number of other street-style blogs rose to prominence, such as *FaceHunter* and *Garance Doré*. But not every blogger shot street style: some chose to photograph themselves, in their own outfits, much as they had done for sites like *The Fashion Spot*. An example is Susie Lau (aka Susie Bubble), who started her blog, *Style Bubble*, in 2006. Using herself as a model brought an extra level of relatability to Susie, and the many others who chose to use themselves as a photographic muse.

By 2009, when Tavi donned her bow, fashion blogging had come of age (though Tavi herself hadn't), and with this new legitimacy fashion bloggers found themselves in the front row at Fashion Week. Magazine editors were not amused, but the fashion industry at large was excited by bloggers and their ability to reach a widespread audience with an immediacy and familiarity that traditional media lacked. This led to an uptick in the value of bloggers, who had previously only been paid in "swag" from brands. Major fashion brands began using them to market fashion in a serious way: Susie Bubble was tapped to model for Gap in 2010, while Scott Schuman created a custom product for Kiehl's in 2011. Agents stepped up to represent these new fashion celebrities: for example, Bryanboy signed with CSA in 2009, and Tavi signed with UTA in 2012. By 2013, Schuman was reportedly making a seven-figure salary just with blog. Fashion blogging had gone from a side project to major media enterprise. In the wake of all this, fashion magazines realized they needed to get serious about

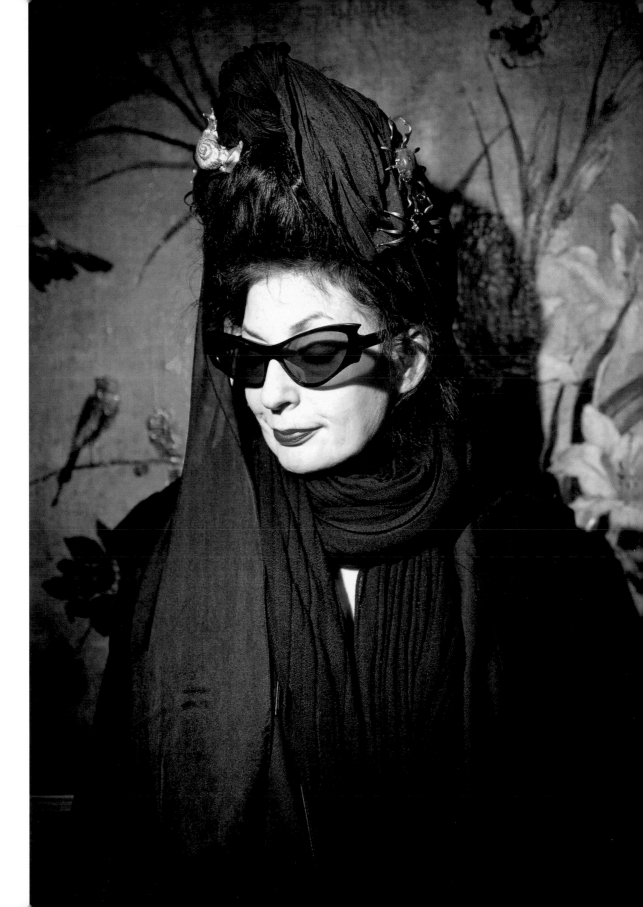

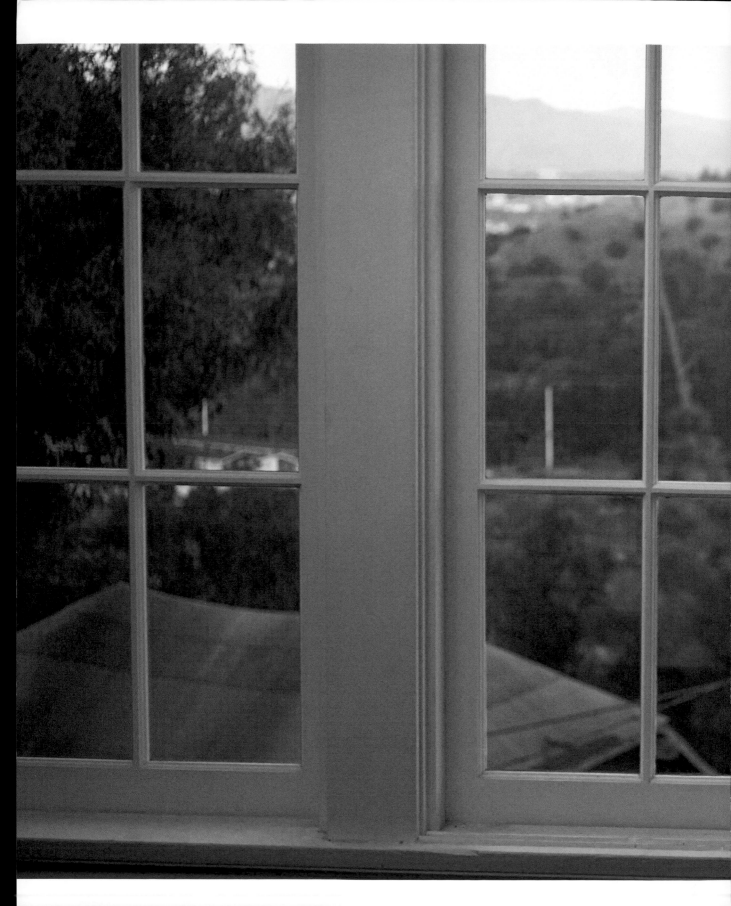

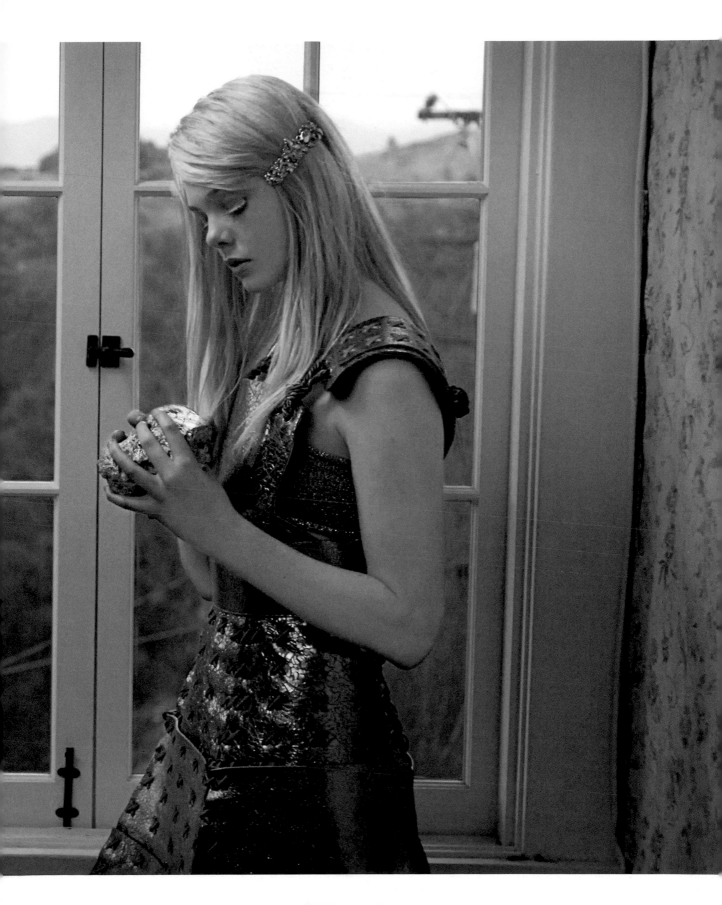

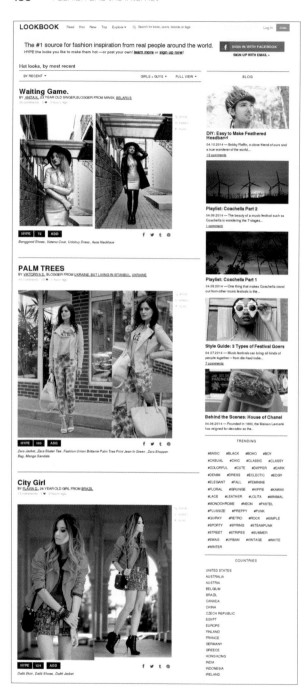

their web presence (see "Fashion Magazines"). Some, like *Dazed & Confused*, brought existing bloggers on board—they tapped Susie Bubble as web editor from 2008 to 2010—while others simply hired editors to manage their own blogs.

As blogs bloomed, fashion became more social. Sites like Lookbook.nu and Chictopia allowed users to sign

left — Fashion goes social on Lookbook.nu, where users can rate each others' style.

up and post photos of their outfits for people to like and comment on; these photos allowed regular people to try out their skills as a stylist and achieve some online fashion clout. The practice of posting style shots online overlapped with the rise of the so-called selfie, self-portraits typically taken with a smartphone and posted to Facebook or, more popularly, Instagram. Selfies gained infamy in 2012, when they were criticized for their attention-seeking like-baiting, but some people posted them for a different reason: to show off their enviable style. On Instagram, when users posted a self-portrait featuring a stylish outfit, they would give it the hashtag #ootd (outfit of the day) to connect with others posting similar photos. But social media wasn't just the territory of fashion amateurs. Industry insiders claimed Twitter and Instagram handles to shore up their social presence (Derek Blasberg maintains extremely successful accounts on both), and live-tweeting runway shows became common practice for fashion editors and bloggers, giving followers instant access to their thoughts on new collections.

Yet it's becoming increasingly unnecessary for people to follow a fashion celebrity live-tweeting a show when they can watch the show themselves, from home. Starting in 2009, when the economic downturn forced fashion houses to adapt to a less ostentatious Fashion Week, designers began to experiment with livestreaming their shows online. First was Louis Vuitton, whose Fall 2009 show was livestreamed on Facebook—then came Alexander McQueen, whose Spring 2010 livestream caused his website to crash after Lady Gaga tweeted it to her followers. By 2012, Prabal Gurung became the first designer to eschew a traditional runway and show his collection by livestream only. Besides making it easier for editors to catch dozens of shows without having to sprint, livestreams have also opened up Fashion Week to a much, much larger audience; designers can show directly to fashion lovers rather than relying on the intermediary of magazines or papers. Despite the clear advantage of being more accessible, livestreams also put more power in the hands of the brands, becoming another form of advertising: with livestreams, they can control the impact of their collection on audiences, rather than relying on the impression they make on more critical fashion editors. Another fashion tool that's unique to the online world is the fashion video, which takes the storylines and aesthetics of traditional fashion editorials and puts them into motion. The most notable player in fashion video is Showstudio.com, founded in November 2000 by fashion photographer Nick Knight, who realized early on that video was the perfect way to show fashion on the internet. Fashion videos quickly became incredibly popular, both as an editorial and advertising tool—prominent brands, realizing the impact of fashion films, began to tap major directors to produce big-budget short films featuring well-known stars. One of the first of these was the *Lady Noir Affair* for Dior, starring Marion Cotillard and directed by Olivier Dahan in 2009; David Lynch directed a later film in the Dior series, called *Lady Blue Shanghai*, also starring Cotillard,

in 2010. As the genre gained popularity, digital storytelling platform Nowness became a launching ground for these cinematic shorts, like Todd Cole's 2011 film for Rodarte, *The Curve of Forgotten Things* (starring Elle Fanning). By 2013, fashion films were popular enough to become fodder for satire, and a mock fashion film starring comedian Lizzy Caplan for Vena Cava went viral with its deft manipulation of the genre's clichés.

Fashion retailing, too, has moved online. One of the earliest and most basic examples is Shopbop, which was founded in 2000 and acquired by Amazon in 2003. Like many e-commerce sites, Shopbop offers thousands of looks that can be purchased from home, any time of the day, and returned if they don't work out. E-commerce has evolved beyond simple online stores, however; some sites, such as Mr. Porter, a men's luxury e-tailer, run custom editorial content that allows a reader to "shop" the stories. And then there's Polyvore, which fuses social media into the mix: it's a user-generated site of fashion collages, which encourages people to sign up and mix/match sets that look much like service-oriented shopping pages in magazines, which readers can then buy from partnered retailers.

Today, it's possible to discover fashion online, buy it there, get feedback on your #ootd, and start your own fashion blog—maybe, in the end, becoming an online fashion celebrity yourself. For any fashion icon wannabe, there's practically no reason to even leave the house... except, of course, to get snapped by a street-style photographer.

Index

Photo Credits

The pictures in this book were graciously made available by the agencies, photographers, and companies mentioned in the credits, or have been taken from the publisher's archive:

p. 8: George Gower (attributed), *Elizabeth I of England*, so-called *Armada Portrait*, circa 1588, Getty Images; p. 10: Hyacinthe Rigaud, *Louis XIV*, 1701, Universal Images Group / Getty Images; p. 11: Élisabeth Vigée Le Brun, *Marie Antoinette*, 1778, Hulton Archive / Imagno / Getty Images; p. 12: Michael Ochs Archives / Getty Images; p. 13: Bates Littlehales / National Geographic / Getty Images; p. 14: Tim Graham / Getty Images; p. 15: Indigo / Getty Images; p. 16: Hulton Archive / Getty Images; p. 17: Gamma-Rapho / Getty Images; p. 18: Lipnitzki / Getty Images; p. 19: Paul Schutzer / Time Life Pictures / Getty Images; p. 21: The Bridgeman Art Library; p. 22: Gordon Parks / Time Life Pictures / Getty Images; p. 24: Niall McInerney; p. 25: AFP / Getty Images; p. 26: Terry O'Neill / Getty Images; p. 27: Hulton Archive / Getty Images; p. 28: Time Life Pictures / Getty Images; p. 30: Popperfoto / Getty Images; p. 31: Paris Match / Getty Images; p. 32: Time Life Pictures/Getty Images; p. 35: WireImage / Getty Images; p. 36: The Bridgeman Art Library; p. 41: Time Life Pictures / Getty Images; p. 42: George Hyningen-Heune, Diana Vreeland Archives; p. 44 left: Ron Galella Collection / WireImage / Getty Images; p. 47: Estate of Martin Munkácsi, Courtesy Howard Greenberg Gallery, New York; p. 49: © Man Ray Trust / ADAGP – Bildkunst / Telimage – 2014; p. 50: © Estate

of Guy Bourdin. Reproduced by permission of Art + Commerce; p. 52: © Juergen Teller; p. 54: Louis Leopold Boilly, *The Singer Chenard, as a Sans-Culotte*, 1792, Giraudon / The Bridgeman Art Library; p. 56: Louis XIV, after 1670, Hulton Archive / Getty Images; p. 57: Ken Welsh / The Bridgeman Art Library; p. 58: PhotoQuest / Getty Images; p. 59: Getty Images; p. 60: Franco Rubartelli / Courtesy Yves Saint Laurent; p. 61: Andy Kropa / Getty Images; p. 62: Getty Images; p. 65: Bernard Boutet de Monvel, *Vous Dites ... Cancan II*, illustration from *La Gazette du Bon Ton*, 1913, The Bridgeman Art Library; p. 67: Gamma-Keystone / Getty Images; p. 68: Sports Illustrated / Getty Images; p. 69: Jonathan Daniel / Getty Images; p. 73: Terry O'Neill / Getty Images; p. 74: Anonymous, *Portrait of Louis XIV Holding a Plan of the Maison Royale de Saint-Cyr*, 17th century, De Agostini / Getty Images; p. 75 left: Robert Dighton, *Portrait of George "Beau" Brummell*, 1805, The Bridgeman Art Library; p. 75 right: J. Russell & Sons / Getty Images; p. 76: Gamma-Rapho / Getty Images; p. 77: Popperfoto / Getty Images; p. 79: Michael Ochs Archives / Getty Images; p. 80: Dimitrios Kambouris / Getty Images for H&M; p. 82: Ian Forsyth / Getty Images; p. 84: Eugene Robert Richee / John Kobal Foundation / Getty Images; p. 85: Michael Webb / Hulton Archive / Getty Images; p. 86: Popperfoto / Getty Images; p. 87: UIG / Getty Images; p. 88: Shelly Gitlow; p. 89: UIG / Getty Images; p. 90: Gamma-Keystone / Getty Images; p. 92: Courtesy of The Advertising Archives; p. 93: Denver Post / Getty Images; pp. 94/95: Courtesy of The Advertising

Archives; p. 97: Sean Gallup / Getty Images; p. 98: UIG / Getty Images; p. 99: Lipnitzki / Roger Viollet / Getty Images; p. 100: Mansell / Mansell / Time Life Pictures / Getty Images; p. 101: Sasha / Hulton Archive / Getty Images; p. 102 left: John Olson / Time Life Pictures / Getty Images; p. 102 right: Denver Post / Getty Images; p. 104: Ebet Roberts / Redferns / Getty Images; p. 105: Larry Busacca / Getty Images; p. 106: Gustav Klimt, Emilie Flöge, 1912, © Wien Museum; p. 109: The Bridgeman Art Library; p. 110: © Les Arts Décoratifs, Paris / Jean Tholance / akg-images; p. 111: © Giacomo Balla / Getty Images; p. 112: The Bridgeman Art Library; p. 113: Gamma-Rapho / Getty; p. 114: Astrid Stawiarz / Getty Images; p. 115: Andrew H. Walker / Getty Images; p. 116: Archive Photos / Getty Images; p. 118: Alfred Eisenstaedt / Time Life Pictures / Getty Images; p. 119: Hulton Archive / Getty Images; p. 120: Paramount Pictures / Photofest; p. 122: Paramount / Everett Collection / Rex Features; p. 123: Columbia Pictures / Sony Pictures Entertainment / Photofest; p. 126: © Deborah Feingold / Corbis; p. 128: Michael Ochs Archives / Getty Images; p. 129: Express / Getty Images; p. 130: GAB Archive / Redferns / Getty Images; p. 131: Richard E. Aaron / Redferns / Getty Images; p. 132: Ebet Roberts / Redferns / Getty Images; p. 133: Steve Pyke / Getty Images; p. 134: WENN Photo Database; p. 135: Kevin Cummins / Getty Images; p. 136: Élisabeth Vigée Le Brun, *Marie Antoinette en chemise*, 1783, akg-images; p. 138: CAP / Roger Viollet / Getty Images; p. 139: Eugene Robert Richee / John Kobal Foundation / Getty Images;

pp. 140/141: Paramount Pictures / Courtesy of Getty Images; p. 142: Jamie McCarthy / WireImage / Getty Images; p. 143: Dimitrios Kambouris / WireImage / Getty Images; p. 145: Michel Dufour / WireImage / Getty Images; p. 147: Reg Lancaster / Hulton Archive / Getty Images; p. 148: DEA Picture Library / De Agostini / Getty Images; p. 149: akg-images; p. 150: © Martin Schoeller / August; p. 151: Fox Photos / Hulton Archive / Getty Images; p. 152: Kevin Winter / Getty Images; p. 153: Stephen Shugerman / Getty Images; p. 154: © Steve Klein for PETA; p. 156: Sasha / Hulton Archive / Getty Images; p. 157: Fred Duval / FilmMagic / Getty Images; p. 159: Handout / Getty Images; p. 160: Dario Cantatore / Getty Images; p. 161: Statia Photography / Getty Images; p. 163: Jewel Samad / AFP / Getty Images; p. 164: *Portrait of Cosimo II de Medici with His Wife and His Son Francesco*, 17th century, De Agostini Picture Library / A. Dagli Orti / The Bridgeman Art Library; p. 166: Chicago History Museum / Getty Images; p. 168: Louise Dahl-Wolfe / © 1989 Center for Creative Photography, Arizona Board of Regents; p. 169: George Stroud / Express / Getty Images; p. 170: Chris Moore / Catwalking / Getty Images; p. 171: Francois Guillot / AFP / Getty Images; p. 173: Pierre Verdy / AFP / Getty Images; p. 174: Jean-Claude Deutsch / Paris Match / Getty Images; p. 175: © Art & commerce / Richard Burbridge; p. 176: © Yuri Manabe; p. 177: Pascal Le Segretain / Getty Images; p. 179: Washington Post / Getty Images; p. 180: Niall McInerney; p. 183: Trago / WireImage / Getty Images; pp. 184/185: © Todd Cole for NOWNESS

Bibliography

Cally Blackman. *100 Years of Fashion*. London, 2012.

Stella Bruzzi. *Undressing Cinema: Clothing and Identity in the Movies*. London, 1997.

Farid Chenoune and Florence Muller. *Yves Saint Laurent*. New York, 2010.

Pamela Church Gibson. *Fashion and Celebrity Culture*. Oxford, 2012.

Elizabeth Cline. *Overdressed: The Shockingly High Cost of Cheap Fashion*. New York, 2010.

Shaun Cole. *Don We Now Our Gay Apparel: Gay Men's Dress in the Twentieth Century*. Oxford, 2000.

Jennifer Craik. *Fashion: The Key Concepts*. New York, 2009.

Joan DeJean. *The Essence of Style: How the French Invented High Fashion, Fine Food, Chic Cafés, Style, Sophistication, and Glamour*. New York, 2005.

Diana De Marly. *The History of Haute Couture, 1850–1950*. New York, 1980.

Elyssa Dimant. *Minimalism and Fashion: Reduction in the Postmodern Era*. New York, 2010.

Regine and Peter W. Engelmeier. *Fashion in Film*. Munich, 1990.

Akiko Fukai et al. *Future Beauty: 30 Years of Japanese Fashion*. London, 2010.

Nancy Hall-Duncan. *The History of Fashion Photography*. New York, 1979.

Dian Hanson. *Terryworld*. Cologne, 2008.

Lisa Immordino Vreeland. *The Eye Has to Travel*. New York, 2011.

Helen Jennings. *New African Fashion*. London, 2011.

Harold Koda and Kohle Yohannan. *The Model as Muse: Embodying Fashion*. New York, 2009.

Janice Miller. *Fashion and Music*. Oxford, 2011.

David Muggleton and Rupert Weinzierl. *The Post-Subcultures Reader*. Oxford, 2004.

John L. Nevinson. *Origin and Early History of the Fashion Plate*. Washington, D.C., 1967.

Alberto Oliva and Norberto Angeletti. *In Vogue: An Illustrated History of the World's Most Famous Fashion Magazine*. New York, 2012.

William Oliver. *Style Feed: The World's Top Fashion Blogs*. London, 2012.

Jane Pavitt. *Fear and Fashion in the Cold War*. London, 2008.

Kerry William Purcell. *Alexey Brodovitch*. London, 2002.

Caroline Rennolds Milbank. *New York Fashion*. New York, 1996.

Ligaya Salazar. *Fashion v Sport*. London, 2008.

Linda M. Scott. *Fresh Lipstick: Redressing Fashion and Feminism*. New York, 2006.

Valerie Steele. *The Berg Companion to Fashion*. Oxford, 2010.

Valerie Steele. *Paris Fashion: A Cultural History*. Oxford, 1998.

Radu Stern. *Against Fashion: Clothing as Art, 1850–1930*. Cambridge, Mass., 2003.

Susan Watkins. *The Public and Private Worlds of Elizabeth I*. London, 1998.

Caroline Weber. *Queen of Fashion: What Marie Antoinette Wore to the Revolution*. New York, 2006.

© Prestel Verlag, Munich · London · New York, 2014

© for the artworks reproduced is held by the artists or photographers, their heirs or assigns, with the exception of: Giacomo Balla © VG Bild-Kunst, Bonn 2014; Guy Bourdin © Estate of Guy Bourdin, Reproduced by permission of Art + Commerce; Man Ray © Man Ray Trust, Paris / VG Bild-Kunst, Bonn 2014; Martin Munkácsi © Estate Martin Munkácsi, Courtesy Howard Greenberg Gallery, New York.

Photo credits: see p. 191

Cover: Audrey Hepburn as Holly Golightly in *Breakfast at Tiffany's* (1961), © Paramount Pictures / Photofest
Back cover: Yves Saint Laurent's "Mondrian" dress (see p. 113); Chanel suits in 1960 (see p. 19); Elizabeth I of England (see p. 8); Manish Arora dress (see p. 173)
Frontispiece: Sarah Burton for Alexander McQueen, Fall/Winter 2012–13 ready-to-wear collection (detail from p. 171)
p. 4: details from pp. 26, 90, 25, 179, 76, 126, 99, 147, 112, 89, 183, 173
p. 6: House of Worth dress, 1883 (detail from p. 166)

Prestel Verlag, Munich
A member of Verlagsgruppe Random House GmbH

Prestel Verlag	Prestel Publishing Ltd.	Prestel Publishing
Neumarkter Strasse 28	14-17 Wells Street	900 Broadway, Suite 603
81673 Munich	London W1T 3PD	New York, NY 10003
Tel. +49 (0)89 4136-0	Tel. +44 (0)20 7323-5004	Tel. +1 (212) 995-2720
Fax +49 (0)89 4136-2335	Fax +44 (0)20 7636-0271	Fax +1 (212) 995-2733
www.prestel.de	www.prestel.com	www.prestel.com

Library of Congress Control Number: 2014940422; British Library Cataloguing-in-Publication Data: a catalogue record for this book is available from the British Library; Deutsche Nationalbibliothek holds a record of this publication in the Deutsche Nationalbibliografie; detailed bibliographical data can be found under: http://www.dnb.de.

Prestel books are available worldwide. Please contact your nearest bookseller or one of the above addresses for information concerning your local distributor.

Editorial direction: Claudia Stäuble
Project management: Julie Kiefer
Picture editor: Dorothea Bethke
Copyediting: Jonathan Fox
Design and layout: Wolfram Söll, designwerk, Munich
Cover design: Corinna Pickart, Munich
Production: Astrid Wedemeyer
Separations: ReproLine Mediateam, Munich
Printing and binding: Druckerei Uhl GmbH & Co. KG, Radolfzell

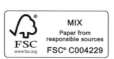

MIX
Paper from responsible sources
FSC® C004229
www.fsc.org

Verlagsgruppe Random House FSC® N001967
The FSC®-certified paper *Hello Fat matt* was supplied by Deutsche Papier Union.

ISBN 978-3-7913-4789-9